Bartosz Gembiak

Testosterone Plan
lifestyle, diet, fertility.

first edition

2023

This book is dedicated to my son, Maciej. May this knowledge help you become the best version of yourself in the future.

Introduction

The life of a modern man is full of challenges. From daily professional duties, through caring for the family, to caring for one's own health and well-being. In this constant rush, it is easy to overlook the signals our body sends us. An improper lifestyle is compounded by toxins, which increasingly poison our bodies every day. This all leads to many problems such as fatigue, lack of energy, concentration problems, and even serious diseases. One of the key elements that determines a man's health is testosterone - a hormone whose improper level can have far-reaching consequences for our well-being and health.

This book is dedicated to all men who want to improve their health and well-being, understand the role that testosterone plays in their lives, and learn how they can affect its level. Regardless of age, health status, or lifestyle, you will find answers to many questions that may bother you. In a simple and accessible way, I explain what are the causes of low testosterone levels, what is its importance for a man's health, how we can improve its natural level, and how to deal with stress, which is one of the most dangerous "enemies" of a healthy lifestyle.

We also discuss issues related to male health in the context of lifestyle diseases, such as infertility, providing knowledge about laboratory tests and treatment methods. We introduce the principles of a healthy diet, emphasizing the role of proper nutrition in maintaining hormonal balance and good mood. You will discover the importance of supplementation for a man's health, learn which supplements are most important for your health and how to use them safely.

Finally, I emphasize the role of physical activity, showing how to exercise properly and effectively to improve your health and well-being. This book is a guide to a healthy lifestyle for a man who wants to enjoy full strength and energy at every stage of life. You will understand how important a role testosterone plays in your life and how you can affect its level to enjoy better health, well-being, and quality of life.

Whether you are a young man who wants to understand how to take care of your health from an early age, or a mature gentleman who wants to improve his well-being and health, this book is for you. You will understand how much your daily habits, diet, physical activity, and supplementation affect your health and well-being. You will learn how to take care of your health to enjoy full strength and energy at every stage of life. It is a compendium of knowledge that will allow you to enjoy better health and well-being, regardless of age.

Table of Contents:

1. Introduction to Men's Health and the Role of Testosterone.

In other words, Some Theory and Research.

Men's health is a broad area that encompasses various aspects, including biology, psychology, and lifestyle. One of the key elements of men's health is the hormone testosterone, which plays a crucial role in regulating many bodily functions and impacts overall well-being and health. Testosterone is the primary male sex hormone, mainly produced in the testes. It is vital for the development of male sexual characteristics and functions, but it also has many other significant roles. Here are a few important aspects regarding the importance of testosterone for men's health:

1. **Impact on physical development**: Testosterone plays a key role in the development of male physical characteristics, such as deep voice, hair growth, and muscle development. It is also responsible for bone development and maintaining bone density.

2. **Regulation of libido and sexual functions**: It influences sexual drive (libido) and regulates sperm production. Low testosterone levels can lead to reduced libido and problems with erection.

3. **Mood and wellbeing regulation**: It influences mood, energy levels, and overall wellbeing. Low testosterone levels can cause fatigue, irritability, depression, and loss of motivation.

4. **Impact on muscle mass and body composition**: It is key to maintaining healthy muscle mass. High testosterone levels

promote building and maintaining muscles, while low levels can lead to muscle loss and increased fat tissue.

5. **Regulation of red blood cell production**: It influences the production of red blood cells in the body. Low testosterone levels can lead to anemia.

6. **Impact on cognitive functions**: Research suggests that testosterone may influence cognitive functions such as memory, focus, and information processing ability.

1.1 Causes of Low Testosterone Levels.

Low testosterone levels in men, also known as hypogonadism, can have many different causes. Here are some of the most common factors that can affect low testosterone levels:

a) **Aging**: One of the natural processes of male aging is the gradual decrease in testosterone levels. As men age, the testicles begin to produce the hormone in smaller amounts, leading to a decrease in testosterone levels in the blood.

b) **Hormonal problems**: Various hormonal problems can affect testosterone production. For example, disorders of the pituitary gland or hypothalamus, which are responsible for regulating hormone production, can lead to lower testosterone levels.

c) **Testicular diseases**: Testicular diseases, such as testicular inflammation, injuries, tumors, or abnormal testicular development, can lead to low testosterone levels.

d) **Obesity**: Overweight and obesity can cause a decrease in testosterone levels. Fat tissue produces the enzyme aromatase, which converts testosterone into estrogens, leading to a decrease in testosterone concentration.

e) **Stress and depression**: Long-term stress and depression can negatively affect the hormonal system and lead to lower testosterone levels.

f) **Tobacco smoking and alcohol abuse**: Smoking and excessive alcohol consumption can have a negative impact on testosterone levels.

g) **Certain medications**: such as anabolic steroids and some painkillers, can lead to lower testosterone levels.

h) **Chronic diseases**: Chronic diseases such as diabetes, kidney disease, liver cirrhosis, or HIV/AIDS, can affect testosterone levels.

i) **Vitamin and mineral deficiency**: A deficiency of certain vitamins and minerals, such as vitamin D and zinc, can affect testosterone production.

1.2 Improving Men's Natural Testosterone Levels:

a) **Healthy diet**: It is important to maintain a balanced diet that provides the right nutrients. Focus on consuming protein, healthy fats (like Omega-3 fats), and vegetables. Additionally, increase the intake of foods rich in zinc (e.g., oysters, cashew nuts, pumpkin seeds) and vitamin D (e.g., fatty fish, eggs, dairy products).

b) **Regular physical activity**: Regular physical exercises, especially strength training, can help boost testosterone levels. Focus on multi-joint exercises like squats, deadlifts, push-ups, which engage multiple muscle groups simultaneously.

c) **Weight control**: Obesity can lead to decreased testosterone levels. If you're overweight, strive to lose weight through a healthy diet and regular physical activity. More on this will be discussed in the subsequent chapters.

d) **Healthy sleep**: Regular and sufficient sleep is important for maintaining a healthy testosterone level. Aim to sleep for 7 to 9 hours each day to provide your body with adequate regeneration.

e) **Stress reduction**: Chronic stress can lead to decreased testosterone levels. Implement relaxation techniques such as meditation, yoga, deep breathing, which will help you reduce stress. An example is the free autogenic training according to Schultz available on YouTube in many forms.

f) **Avoiding alcohol and smoking**: Excessive alcohol consumption and smoking can have a negative impact on testosterone levels. Try to limit alcohol consumption and avoid smoking.

g) **Avoiding excessive physical stress**: Overloading the body, such as long-term high-intensity training, can lead to a decrease in testosterone levels. Ensure you have enough time to rest and regenerate between workouts.

h) **Supplementation**: In some cases, with low testosterone levels, a doctor may recommend testosterone supplementation. However, the decision about supplementation should be made by a doctor after proper assessment and diagnosis. Testosterone Replacement Therapy, described in later chapters.

From the above contents, the following conclusions can be drawn: the correct level of testosterone in a man is crucial for his proper functioning in virtually every area of life. Its condition has a key impact on health, and a proper, stable lifestyle results in its optimal level.

1.3 Stress as a Catalyst for Health Destruction.

There is no way not to mention stress here as a factor initiating all negative transformations in the body. Stress is a common experience in everyday life and can have both short-term and long-term health consequences. It has a huge impact on health:

a) **Hormonal system**: It can affect the hormonal system, including the level of cortisol, often referred to as the stress hormone. Chronic stress can lead to excessive cortisol secretion, which can disrupt hormonal balance, including lowering testosterone levels. Low testosterone can lead to decreased libido, muscle mass reduction, mood deterioration, and fatigue.

b) **Mental health**: Chronic stress can affect men's mental health. It can cause problems such as depression, anxiety, fatigue, irritability, and difficulty concentrating. Men often tend to hold back emotions and mask their stress, which can lead to long-term mental burden.

c) **Heart disease**: Chronic stress can increase the risk of developing heart disease in men. High cortisol levels can affect cholesterol levels and blood pressure, as well as lead to changes in the vascular system that may contribute to heart disease.

d) **Immune system**: It can affect the immune system, weakening it and making you more susceptible to infections and diseases. Chronic stress can affect the body's ability to fight infections and cause chronic inflammation.

e) **Sleep problems**: It can lead to difficulties with sleep, such as insomnia or irregular sleep. Improper sleep can have a negative impact on men's physical and mental health, affecting energy levels, mood, and the ability to concentrate.

1.4 How to Cope with Stress?

First and foremost, it's important to realize that humans are the only organisms on Earth that can induce stress - a disease - with their thoughts. Just as our thoughts can influence the negative state of our health, we can also improve our health. This can be done through practicing relaxation techniques such as meditation, deep breathing, and yoga. Physical activity can also help in stress reduction by triggering the release of endorphins - the happiness hormones. It is important to maintain a healthy diet, find emotional support, converse with loved ones or seek help from specialists. Ensure that you rest and sleep regularly, maintaining a healthy sleep schedule. Identify a GOAL - a hobby or activity that brings you joy and relaxation. Avoid excessive intake of caffeine, alcohol, and other substances that can intensify stress.

A topic seldom discussed in the context of stress and health is relationships. Although this guide doesn't strictly address the topic of relationships, it's worth noting that it often plays a crucial role in this context.

Scientists from the University of Utah (USA) have found that men who are in a marital relationship tend to live almost 10 years longer than others. Feminists often refer to these studies and take them out of context. The studies indicate that married men live longer, but also men who are not married but have a higher education live longer. These studies completely overlooked the fact of divorced men (who were in marriages) and they statistically live shorter lives. Not to mention, the majority of suicides among men are committed in the context of a relationship with a woman. So, what can be concluded from these studies? Men who lead stable lives, free from excessive emotionality, live longer both in a relationship and outside of it. However, in a marital relationship, there is a risk of divorce, up to 23% annually (statistical data from Poland). So, it's like playing Russian roulette and each year we're putting one bullet into the chamber of a revolver, with one of the four chambers presenting the risk. Evaluate this risk yourselves. Divorce for a man is usually a massive stress (only greater stress is associated with the death of a spouse) and it can have health and financial consequences for many years.

1.4.1 Subconscious Programming for Happiness.

Indeed, "programming the subconscious for happiness" is a very effective and lasting method of getting rid of stress. Fighting stress with affirmations can be an effective strategy. It's crucial that the affirmation is based on real aspects of our life. We use statements in it, not goals: For example, "I own my own apartment", not "I want to own my own apartment". Only 3-4 examples are sufficient for affirmations, which we then repeat to ourselves.

Here are some examples of affirmations that can help with stress management:

1. I own my own apartment / house.

2. I have a stable job.

3. I can count on my parents.

4. I have healthy children.

5. I have money (in the sense that I am secure, nothing threatens me, having security in the form of money must be real)

6. I have a pension.

7. I can handle any situation.

8. I am well educated, I have many skills, and I will always find a job.

9. I am slim (this is an example of an affirmation when starting the "weight loss" process. The subconscious will do everything to live up to our affirmation.)

10. I am happy (this is an example of my favorite affirmation, it's worth doing it right after waking up).

Affirmations should be repeated regularly and spoken with conviction. They can be used in various situations, such as upon waking in the morning, when returning home from work, or before sleep. Affirmations alone won't solve problems (although through programming the subconscious), the subconscious tries to solve them without our logical will.

It is also important to take actions that will help reduce stress, such as meditation, physical activity, maintaining a good diet, and a healthy lifestyle. Regularly repeated affirmations yield spectacular results and can also introduce permanent change in our body.

As one can easily realize, we often unintentionally program our subconscious negatively. An example of such an affirmation is "I'm stupid", "I'm unlucky". It should be noted that we are also subconsciously programmed by the media. An ideal example of this is television advertising (if it didn't work and didn't increase sales, no one would spend money on it) or the dumbing down of society through mass media. It is worth filtering news and being aware that everything you let into your thoughts in some way affects you..

Revisiting the past associated with trauma only subconsciously strengthens and reinforces negative and stressful thoughts each time, and since the past cannot be changed, there is no point in going back to it. Worrying about the future also makes no sense, as it is uncertain. Often, building negative scenarios only deepens stress, and instead of wasting energy, it is worth taking action in the present to mitigate negative future scenarios.

An interesting feature of the mind is action, or rather its impact on reducing fear. Therefore, setting goals and realizing them through action is important. The conclusion is that we need to be vigilant about the impact of negative affirmations and media on our subconscious programming. Avoiding returning to the past and worrying about the future allows us to focus on the present and create positive scenarios. Action is key to reducing fear and achieving success. Taking control of our mind and consciously programming positive beliefs can contribute to improving the quality of life, and therefore building our happiness.

1.5 Causes of Infertility in Men.

At this point, it should be noted that infertility clinics do not treat male infertility. In fact, basic tests for men are not even conducted there. Apart from semen tests, which are expensive and are meant to prove infertility. The clinics draw the largest profits from in vitro procedures and the entire admission and care process for a couple is reduced to this.

Everything is already known about female fertility and infertility, while male fertility is completely not talked about. It is marginalized because sperm is cheap. One man can impregnate hundreds of thousands of women, so the quality of male sperm is not perceived as a global problem. A doctor cannot provide an answer as to why a particular man is infertile - unless it comes to obvious cases, such as congenital defects. What's more, as I already mentioned, the infertility clinic will be proving your irreversible infertility, even though you have already had children before. And no, this is not a joke on my part, but a verified procedure.

The most significant factors indicated as the reason for the inability to conceive a child are:

a) **Low sperm quality**: One of the main factors of male infertility is low sperm quality, that is, a low number of sperm, their abnormal shape or mobility. This can result from various factors such as infections, hormonal disorders, testicular damage, improper sperm production, or the use of certain medications.

b) **Hormonal disorders**: Such as hypothyroidism, hyperpituitarism, testosterone deficiency, or an excess of estrogens, can affect sperm production and quality.

c) **Congenital anatomical defects**: Some men may have congenital anatomical defects such as blocked sperm pathways, abnormal testicle placement, or abnormalities in the structure of the vas deferens. These defects can interfere with sperm transport.

d) **Sexually transmitted diseases**: Sexually transmitted infections such as chlamydia, gonorrhea, or human papillomavirus (HPV) can lead to damage to the vas deferens, which can affect fertility.

e) **Reproductive system diseases**: Such as orchitis, epididymitis, or varicocele, can affect sperm production and quality.

f) **Environmental factors**: They can have a negative impact on male fertility. Examples include exposure to toxic substances, ionizing radiation, smoking, excessive alcohol or drug consumption.

g) **Problems with erection and ejaculation**: Some health problems, such as erectile dysfunction or premature ejaculation, can make it difficult to get pregnant.

And if you don't have congenital anatomical defects, all other factors come down to the man's health. Once upon a time, I came across studies (unfortunately, I am not able to find them), which suggested that male fertility, like female fertility, is periodic. Generally, it is assumed that a healthy man can conceive a child practically until old age or even until death. The theory of the periodicity of male fertility could also be confirmed by the above-mentioned reasons for low testosterone levels. So, for example, stress could exclude the periodic fertility of a man, by disturbing the hormonal system. Interestingly, it could exclude alcohol abuse and poor diet – because as it is widely known, pathology has the most children, and therefore is the most fertile. At this point, a bold theory could be put forward that it is an excess of food, not its lack, that increases infertility, but this topic will be described in the following chapters on diet.

2. Laboratory Tests and Treatment.

All efforts to maintain proper health should begin with laboratory tests. Of course, the most important feature of these is the level of testosterone. However, not only should it be determined, because other hormones indirectly affect the level of testosterone. In addition, with each test, a general blood morphology should also be performed, as it can detect other abnormalities and perform more detailed tests.

So, what should a man test to get to know the image of his health norms:

- **General morphology** (reference norms are found on the result card and can be taken literally)
- **TESTOSTERONE** (norms defined in the next chapter)
- **SHBG** (20-110 nmol/l)
- **LH** (1,70 – 8,60 mIU/ml)
- **FSH** (1,5-12,4 uIU/ml)
- **PROLACTIN** (4,0-15,2 ng/ml)
- **TSH + fT4** (TSH should be about 1.5 uIU/ml, although its normal reference value is in the range of 0.27-4.2 uIU/ml, while the value of fT4 should be 1.5-1.7 ng/dl, although the correct reference value is marked 0.93-1.7 mg/dl)

and recommended additional tests - once, for verification:

- **ALT** (below 40 units per liter (U/L))
- **ESR** (below 15 mm/h)
- **Glucose** (fasting 70-99 mmol/l)

In this section, I intentionally omitted cholesterol tests, the lipid profile, for two reasons. The first one is the controversy over setting norms and its impact on health, and the second, more important one – a proper diet and exercise regimen will 100% effectively lower cholesterol – which I will discuss in the following chapters.

Testosterone – is a hormone that influences our appearance, sexual functions, muscle work, and behavior. Moreover, it's also responsible for increasing the production of red blood cells in the bone marrow, which is important for the transport of oxygen to the brain. Regular testing of testosterone levels in men is recommended from the age of 16-17 and should be conducted once a year. As part of a blood sample examination, it's crucial to monitor two factors - free and total testosterone. It's worth noting that the level of testosterone tends to decrease with age, and its concentration can be influenced by various factors such as stress, environmental pollution, or diet. It's also crucial to monitor the concentration of SHBG protein (sex hormone-binding globulin), as an abnormal concentration of total testosterone may result from disorders in the synthesis of this protein. Examination of SHBG protein concentration can provide valuable information in the context of testosterone level evaluation. To obtain accurate information about the testosterone level and interpretation of test results, it's always recommended to consult with a specialist doctor who can accurately assess the situation and provide appropriate advice.

LH – (luteinizing hormone) plays a significant role in diagnosing infertility and impotence in men. The LH concentration in men's blood is measured simultaneously with the testosterone level. An elevated LH concentration may indicate primary testicular failure, just like a reduced testosterone level. Conversely, high LH levels and elevated testosterone may indicate androgen insensitivity syndrome. If the LH concentration is low and is accompanied by a decrease in testosterone level, this may indicate secondary testicular failure, which may be caused by disorders of the pituitary gland or hypothalamus. Low luteinizing hormone and elevated testosterone levels may occur in individuals taking exogenous testosterone. A low LH level can also indicate testicular cancer, although it should be remembered that this is just one possibility and requires further diagnosis. In the case of interpreting the results of LH and testosterone tests and diagnosing the above conditions, it is always recommended to consult with a specialist doctor who can accurately assess the situation and adjust appropriate treatment.

FSH – (follicle-stimulating hormone) is a hormone responsible for the maturation of ovarian follicles in women and sperm in men. FSH concentration measurement is used in the diagnosis of infertility, impotence, menstrual disorders, and puberty. FSH hormone is one of the gonadotropins synthesized by the beta cells of the anterior pituitary. It plays a key role in the development and maintenance of gonadal tissue functions, which are responsible for the production and release of steroid hormones. In men, measuring FSH concentration can provide information about testicular function and sperm production. Elevated FSH levels in men may suggest spermatogenesis disorders or testicular insufficiency.

Prolactin – is a hormone that is significant both in women and men. In men, prolactin stimulates the testes to produce testosterone, is responsible for sexual functions, and supports the functioning of the immune system. Reference values for prolactin concentration in men are usually lower than 15 ng/ml. However, it should be noted that the test result may be influenced by stress and the time since the last meal. Low prolactin in men may be associated with erection and ejaculation problems, as well as decreased androgen levels and semen quality. Conversely, high prolactin concentration in men, known as hyperprolactinemia, can negatively affect libido, lead to the onset of gynecomastia (enlargement of breasts in men), and increase the risk of osteoporosis.

TSH is a pituitary hormone that oversees the work of the thyroid; fT4 is a hormone produced directly by the thyroid. The interdependencies between the concentrations of these hormones allow the diagnosis of primary or secondary disorders of hyperactivity or hypothyroidism. These disorders are associated with a direct impact on metabolism (respectively weight loss or weight gain, dry skin or excessive sweating, constipation or diarrhea), synthesis of SHBG protein, semen quality (change in quantity and mobility of sperm), fertility, and emotional balance.

ALT (alanine aminotransferase), also known as alanine transaminase, is an enzyme mainly present in liver cells. It is important in assessing liver function and diagnosing various liver diseases. Elevated ALT levels may indicate liver damage, such as viral hepatitis (e.g., hepatitis A, B, C), toxic liver damage (e.g., due to alcohol abuse or use of certain medications), fatty liver disease, autoimmune liver disease, or even liver cancer. However, it's worth remembering that the result of elevated ALT activity alone is not a specific indicator of a particular liver disease. For an accurate diagnosis and determination of the cause of elevated ALT levels, additional tests and consultation with a specialist, such as a gastroenterologist or hepatologist, are usually required.

ESR (Erythrocyte Sedimentation Rate), is a marker used in medical diagnostics to assess the presence and severity of an inflammatory state in the body. ESR measurement involves determining the rate at which red blood cells settle in a tube specifically designed for this purpose. Under normal conditions, red blood cells settle at the bottom of the tube due to gravity. However, in the presence of an inflammatory state, such as infection or autoimmune disease, proteins called fibrinogen, which are present in the blood, can stick together, causing increased blood viscosity. As a result, red blood cells settle more slowly, leading to an increase in the ESR. The ESR result is given in millimeters per hour (mm/h) and is interpreted in the context of other clinical symptoms of the patient. Higher ESR values may indicate the presence of an inflammatory state, but they do not indicate a specific cause. Therefore, it's important to conduct additional tests and evaluate other laboratory parameters for an accurate diagnosis. It should be noted that ESR is a non-specific indicator and can also be elevated in other states, such as cancer, rheumatoid arthritis, aortic aneurysm, or kidney disease. Conversely, some factors, such as anemia, can lower the ESR result.

Fasting plasma glucose (also known as fasting blood sugar) is a measurement of the concentration of glucose in the blood after at least 8 hours of fasting, i.e., from the time of the last meal. It is one of the basic tests used to assess blood sugar levels and diagnose carbohydrate metabolism disorders, especially diabetes.

Normal fasting glucose levels usually range between 70 and 100 milligrams per deciliter (mg/dl) or 3.9 to 5.6 millimoles per liter (mmol/l). Here are the approximate ranges for fasting glucose levels:
 • Normoglycemia (normal fasting glucose level): 70-100 mg/dl (3.9-5.6 mmol/l)
 • Prediabetes: 100-125 mg/dl (5.6-6.9 mmol/l)

• Diabetes: 126 mg/dl (7.0 mmol/l) or higher

Fasting glucose levels above 126 mg/dl (7.0 mmol/l) in two or more independent measurements suggest the occurrence of diabetes. However, a single high result may require confirmation with additional tests.

Abnormal concentrations of these hormones can be responsible for ineffective spermatogenesis and consequently poor semen parameters, difficulties in conceiving offspring, erectile problems, but also for lowered mood, and even depression. With the result of the first detailed examinations, regardless of whether they are within the laboratory norm or not, one should visit a primary care physician and ask for a referral to an endocrinologist. It is also possible to directly privately visit an endocrinologist but only one whose reviews we have checked on the internet, as even privately practicing endocrinologists can treat in a template manner, contrary to medical art

2.1. Testosterone Norms.

It's important to start here with testosterone norms for women. Usually, a test for the correct level of free testosterone is ordered when the total testosterone level is questionable.

Testosterone norms in women can vary slightly depending on the laboratory performing the test and the woman's age. However, the general reference ranges for testosterone in women, globally accepted, are typically:

Total testosterone:

• Prepubertal girls: below 20 ng/dl (nanograms per deciliter)

Adult women:

• Before menopause: 15-70 ng/dl

• After menopause: 0-55 ng/dl

Free testosterone:

• Before menopause: 0.1-6.4 ng/dl

• After menopause: 0.1-2.7 ng/dl

However, it should be noted that testosterone levels can vary depending on the phase of the menstrual cycle in women, as well as from individual body characteristics.

Testosterone norms in men can also vary slightly depending on the laboratory performing the test. Usually, a test for the correct level of free testosterone is ordered when the total testosterone level is questionable.

Below are the general reference ranges for testosterone in men, globally accepted:

Total testosterone:

Adult men:

• Age 19-39 years: 264-916 ng/dl (nanograms per deciliter)

• Age 40-59 years: 198-890 ng/dl

• Age 60-69 years: 156-819 ng/dl

• Age over 70 years: 113-753 ng/dl

Free testosterone:

Adult men:

• Age 19-39 years: 9.3-26.5 pg/ml (picograms per milliliter)

• Age 40-59 years: 6.5-22.9 pg/ml

• Age 60-69 years: 5.0-19.0 pg/ml

• Age over 70 years: 4.4-16.8 pg/ml

However, it's worth remembering that these standards are general and can vary depending on individual body characteristics and the methodology used in the laboratory.

In Poland, the standard testosterone range **for men** is between 9.0 and 34.7 nmol/l (260–1000 ng/dl), and for women, it is between 0.52 and 2.43 nmol/l (15–70 ng/dl). Additionally, it is generally accepted that a level below 8 nmol/l in men requires substitution, that is, supplementation through the intake of pharmacological preparations. From the above standards, we can establish a conversion factor of 1 nmol/l $\cong$ 28.84 ng/dl. This means that the testosterone level in men can be as much as 66.66 times higher than in women according to the Polish standard. For this reason, it is generally accepted that men, on average, have a sexual drive that is 4 times higher than women. Consequently, this need takes on a completely different character in men and women. A man with the testosterone level of a woman would practically be deprived of sexual drive.

Studies suggest that testosterone levels in men have been gradually decreasing since about the middle of the 20th century. For example, an analysis of data from a study conducted on men in the United States from 1987-2004 showed an average decrease in testosterone levels of about 1% per year. However, it should be noted that there is no clear answer to the question of exact testosterone levels in previous generations, as studies in this area are relatively limited and differ depending on the population studied and the methodology. Following this line of thought – taking the year 1950 as the baseline level of testosterone in men, by the year 2020, this level was 70% higher than that assumed in the current standards. Therefore, the standards **for men** would look like this - for men, it is between **15.3 and 58.99 nmol/l (442–1700 ng/dl)**, so the average level of normal testosterone **would be 37.15 nmol/l (1071 ng/dl)**. As you can see, the standard testosterone level for a man is practically the level of the current upper limit of testosterone standards for men. Therefore, it should be accepted that our testosterone should reach the current upper limit of the standard.

2.2 Adverse High Testosterone.

High levels of testosterone in men are also not beneficial. They can lead to various health problems. Here are some potential consequences:

a) **Aggression and uncontrolled behavior**: High levels of testosterone can lead to increased aggression and uncontrolled behavior. Individuals with high testosterone levels may be more prone to anger outbursts and have more difficulty controlling their emotions.

b) **Sleep problems**: High testosterone levels can affect sleep quality and lead to insomnia or irregular sleep patterns. This can result in fatigue and lack of energy during the day, which, over the long term, affects brain degeneration.

c) **Increased risk of cardiovascular diseases:** Research suggests that high testosterone levels can increase the risk of cardiovascular diseases, such as atherosclerosis, high blood pressure, and heart attack. However, this relationship is not yet fully understood and requires further research.

d) **Propensity for baldness:** High testosterone levels can contribute to premature baldness in some men. Testosterone is converted into dihydrotestosterone (DHT), which can shorten the hair life cycle and cause hair loss.

e) **Fertility problems:** Paradoxically, although testosterone is a key male hormone, an excess of this hormone can negatively affect fertility. High testosterone levels can lead to decreased sperm production or disturbances in sperm quality.

Of course, excessively high testosterone levels do not occur naturally, they are most often associated with administering its variants orally or through injections. It is important that testosterone supplementation is carried out under medical supervision and in accordance with a doctor's recommendations. Long-term use of large doses of testosterone without proper medical control can lead to serious and irreversible health complications. Therefore, Testosterone Replacement Therapy should be considered a last resort, after exhausting natural ways to increase it.

2.3 Testosterone Replacement Therapy.

Testosterone Replacement Therapy (TRT) is a medical procedure in which men with low testosterone levels are given testosterone supplementation to restore appropriate hormone levels. TRT is used when men have a testosterone deficiency, which can lead to symptoms and health problems

Testosterone Replacement Therapy can bring various benefits to men who suffer from testosterone deficiency. Here are some of the potential benefits of TRT:

a) **Improvement in libido and sexual functions:** Low testosterone levels can lead to a decrease in libido and erectile dysfunction. TRT can help restore sexual abilities and improve sex life.

b) **Mood improvement:** Low testosterone levels can affect mood, causing irritability, depression, fatigue, and lack of motivation. TRT can help improve mood and overall well-being.

c) **Increase in muscle mass and strength:** Testosterone plays a role in building and maintaining muscle mass. Testosterone replacement therapy can contribute to an increase in muscle mass and strength, especially in men who exercise regularly.

d) **Improvement in bone density:** Low testosterone levels can lead to loss of bone mass and an increased risk of osteoporosis. TRT can help improve bone density and reduce the risk of fractures.

e) **Improvement in energy levels and endurance**: Testosterone deficiency can lead to feelings of fatigue, decreased energy, and limited endurance. Testosterone replacement therapy can help restore energy levels and improve overall endurance.

It's important that testosterone replacement therapy is conducted under the supervision of a doctor and according to medical recommendations. The doctor can conduct the appropriate tests and assess whether TRT is suitable for a specific patient. Improper use of TRT or abuse of testosterone can lead to serious health problems. Unfortunately, in Poland, there are still few doctors specifically dealing with TRT, and specialists of this type are most often available in provincial cities. Theoretically, any endocrinologist can carry out TRT. However, it is worth checking the opinion of each doctor to whom we intend to report for Testosterone Replacement Therapy.

It is important to treat TRT as a last resort when other methods have not yielded results. Administering TRT under the supervision of a doctor and according to appropriate recommendations is usually safe and effective. However, there are some potential risks and side effects associated with testosterone replacement therapy. Here are some factors to consider:

- **Increased risk of cardiovascular diseases**: Some studies suggest that TRT may increase the risk of cardiovascular diseases, such as heart attack and stroke, especially in older men or those with existing heart conditions. However, other studies do not confirm this connection, so further research is necessary in this field.

- **Increased risk of blood clots**: TRT may increase the risk of blood clots forming, especially in men with existing risk factors for thrombosis, such as obesity or smoking. If symptoms of a blood clot appear, such as leg pain, shortness of breath, or chest pain, you should contact a doctor immediately.

- **Increased risk of prostate enlargement**: TRT may lead to further growth of the prostate in men with existing prostate enlargement (BPH). In such cases, careful monitoring of the prostate condition during therapy is necessary.

- **Decreased production of your own testosterone**: Regular administration of external testosterone during TRT can lead to a decrease in the production of endogenous (own) testosterone by the testicles. Therefore, when considering TRT, it is necessary to understand and discuss potential side effects in detail and the need to monitor testosterone levels during therapy.

- **Changes in blood clotting**: TRT can affect blood composition, including the number of red blood cells and hematocrit. In case of excessive increase in hematocrit (increased concentration of red blood cells), there is a risk of blood thickening, which can lead to health problems. Regular blood monitoring is important during TRT.

3. The Role of Diet in Maintaining Healthy Testosterone Levels.

Virtually no one today questions the effects of taking medications. Doctors prescribe a specific drug for a specific ailment, and often we can see for ourselves that the orally administered drug works in a certain way on our bodies.

So why do so few people believe in diet and that what we eat has a direct impact on our bodies?

Possibly the answer to this question lies in the fact that food is not as concentrated as drugs and its effect on the body is weaker and more spread out over time. However, this does not change the fact that what we eat, how we eat, and when we eat has a crucial impact on our health. In my opinion, more than any other cause.

If we put diesel in a petrol car or vice versa, the car will stop working properly very quickly. The human body operates slightly differently, it's more complex, so the wrong fuel in the form of food "damages" the body in a cunningly slow way, thereby giving us the impression that it has little effect on our health.

There are numerous types of diets and theories on this topic. In this chapter, I will try to introduce just a few of them. Finally, I will present my own diet, which was developed based on medical knowledge and personal experience with diets.

In addition to strictly defined diets, I will also describe one-off therapies that can have a positive impact on the functioning of the body, such as silicon therapy, or information about the impact of plastic on the body.

3.1 The Diet that will Ruin Your Life.

The diet that will surely ruin your life is the traditional diet, i.e., a systematic few meals in amounts from 3 to 5. Why? You will find out about this only if you read this entire chapter. If the answer to this question were simple, probably everyone would know about it, and I wouldn't need to discuss it.

In a nutshell, it can be assumed that an excess of food is more responsible for diseases than its deficiency. However, a moderate deficiency is basically a recipe for health. Many diseases (like heart disease) did not occur until the second half of the 20th century. As you may have read from the chapter dedicated to testosterone, its gradual decrease in men by one percent per year also began to occur from the mid-20th century. Since then, the way of eating, its quality, and quantity have changed. In the past, to eat a carrot, you had to first plant it yourself, then you had to leave the house to pick it up, bring it home, and then eat it. Meat was even more difficult to access, and food itself was much less processed. In addition to this, food was generally much more expensive due to technologically poor agriculture, less efficient and more costly transport, primitive food storage and preservation technology, and limited international trade. The vast majority of human work involved physical labor, even simple housework, without electrification (such as laundry) cost incomparably more energy than it does today. Based on this, it can be concluded that there is a correlation between physical exertion - the quantity and quality of food consumed, and health.

The idea of promoting multiple meals throughout the day likely supports improving the economy. It is therefore beneficial for the economy. The pharmaceutical industry also doesn't necessarily prioritize human health, as it is often ranked as the 2nd or 3rd most profitable sector of the global economy.

At this point, it's worth mentioning statins. Statins are a group of drugs used to lower blood cholesterol levels. Cholesterol is a fatty compound present in the body. Statins are one of the most profitable branches of the pharmaceutical industry. The cholesterol level at which statin treatment is recommended has been directly established to maximize profits from their sales, so that the largest possible group of people "fall into" statin treatment. Moreover, we already know today that statins do not in any way save health. In fact, after reading the leaflet of any statins available on the market, any reasonable person would not take them, if only for the fact that statins destroy muscles. In the chapter devoted to the tests that a man should perform, I deliberately omitted the topic related to cholesterol, because there are very simple ways to lower it. In addition, the diet I propose over a longer period of time (several months) guarantees a proper cholesterol level.

And now the best part, for the entirety of human science today, it is accepted that scientific studies are repeatable in 60% of cases. In exact sciences, such as mathematics and physics, the repeatability of studies is nearly 100%. In sciences like psychology, it's only 33%. However, the most dishonest science are medical studies. "For example, it has been shown that medical studies in the area of cancer are repeatable only in 10% of cases [Begley 2013]" I think this information doesn't require a comment.

3.2 Diet, Why It's Hard to Start.

Each of us associates a diet with sacrifices. Indeed, if you have never cared about what you eat or have been eating according to some unhealthy pattern that has become your habit, or worse, if you eat random dishes or only what you like, then changing your eating habit will be a challenge, especially of a mental nature.

Except for the case in which you want to quickly improve your health, your diet should become a new habit. So we are not talking about a diet for something specific, but about healthy eating habits for life. Otherwise, we face a return "to crime" and a "yo-yo" effect

Here are a few factors that may make starting a diet difficult:

○ **Lack of motivation**: One of the main reasons for difficulty in starting a diet is a lack of sufficient motivation. A diet requires a change in eating habits and approach to food, which can be hard to accept and implement. Lack of motivation can lead to resistance or discouragement.

○ **Lack of a plan and goals**: A proper start to a diet requires a clear action plan and setting specific goals. Without such structure and goals, it is easy to get distracted or postpone starting until later.

○ **Addiction to unhealthy food**: If you're used to consuming unhealthy food, such as fast food, sweets, or processed products, it may be hard to break these habits and start a healthy diet. Addiction to such food can lead to strong cravings and difficulties in replacing it with healthier alternatives.

o **Difficulty in meal planning and preparing healthy dishes**: Not planning meals and a lack of skills in preparing healthy dishes can make starting a diet difficult. A lack of time or cooking skills can lead to resorting to quick, unhealthy options.

o **Lack of social support**: A diet can be hard, especially when you don't have the support of family, friends, or a partner. This often comes with social pressure, temptations, and difficulties in maintaining healthy habits when your environment does not support your choice.

o **Emotional eating:** Often, eating is associated with emotions, such as stress, sadness, or boredom. Some people turn to food as a form of comfort or a way to cope with emotions. Breaking these emotional eating habits can be difficult and requires awareness and alternative strategies for dealing with emotions.

In my opinion, the hardest part is making the decision itself. Often it takes many weeks. For people who love to eat and have never had any experience with restricting food, this may seem like a very difficult task. It would be good for everyone to ask themselves at this point: What do you prefer, to undergo surgery in the future, suffer from a serious illness, or introduce some healthy habits into your life, which over time will seem like something completely normal, as it is currently in my case. I could compare introducing a diet into my life to learning to drive a car. In the beginning, both the rules and the practice seem incredibly difficult, but later, when you have had your driving license for a few years, it seems completely normal.

It takes a maximum of 66 days for something to become a habit. So, we're talking about 2 months of "hardship". What the research says - the time needed to form habits can vary for different people and depends on many factors. It is suggested that implementing a new habit can take from about 21 to 66 days.

Studies conducted by University College London suggest that on average it takes about 66 days for a new action to become automated and become a habit. However, the results of these studies are varied and there is no definite number of days that works for everyone. The time needed to form a habit can depend on the following factors:

- **Individual differences**: Each person has a different learning and adaptation pace. The time needed to form a habit can vary depending on individual traits and predispositions.

- **Difficulty of the habit**: Some habits are easier to form than others. If the habit is complicated or requires more effort, it may take longer to become automatic.

- **Regularity of practice**: The frequency of performing a particular activity can affect how quickly a habit is formed. Regularly practicing a new habit can speed up the process.

- **Motivation and determination**: Strong motivation and determination can help form a habit faster. If you are motivated and consistent, you are more likely to maintain the habit for a longer period of time.

3.3 Diet by Ewa Dąbrowska.

I started my adventure with dieting from Dr. Ewa Dąbrowska's diet when I was having serious back problems. I stumbled upon this diet completely by chance. In a very simplified version, it's a fruit and vegetable diet. At that time, I considered fruits and vegetables more as weeds than "serious" food. My problems started after I turned 30 and over the following years they led me to problems with putting on my underwear while standing up. With recurring episodes of pain, lasting 3 weeks, during which I was taking several types of oral painkillers. At some point, I ended up with a doctor who specialized in spine surgeries and I was scheduled for a surgery appointment. Thanks to this diet, the operation did not take place and today I only feel mild pain associated with consuming sweets. It happens sporadically and at my own request, because I know the cause of the pain – yes, it is a high dose of sugar, consumed over a period of 2-3 days.

It's worth mentioning here that not only during that period was I suffering from back pain, but I also had a disrupted hormonal system, which I found out about a few years later. The only cause of my health condition was a random diet and chronic stress related to divorce and breakups, so what I wrote about earlier. Stress has a huge impact on men's health. A stable relationship has a positive impact on health, while a turbulent one - the stress associated with it - destroys as powerfully as a malignant tumor.

During that period, Dr. Dąbrowska's diet was the only known healing diet, which I could not believe myself. At this point, it's necessary to introduce the profile of Ewa Dąbrowska.

Dr. Ewa Dąbrowska is a Polish doctor and specialist in the field of functional medicine and dietetics. She is also an author of books and conducts popular health programs. Her approach to health is based on a holistic view that includes both physical and emotional and social aspects.

Dr. Ewa Dąbrowska is best known for developing a vegetable-fruit diet, also called the vegetable-fruit diet according to Dr. Ewa Dąbrowska. This diet is based on eating mainly raw vegetables, fruits, juices, and vegetable soups. It is recommended to avoid meat products, dairy, cereals, processed food, as well as alcohol and coffee. According to Dr. Ewa Dąbrowska, this diet has a beneficial effect on body detoxification and health improvement. In her medical practice, Dr. Ewa Dąbrowska applies a therapeutic approach that includes not only diet but also lifestyle changes, physical activity, movement therapy, supplementation, body cleansing, and emotional support. Her approach focuses on nutrition that supports health and restores the body's balance.

Interestingly, the diet has followers among the people who use it. This can be seen, for example, on the Facebook and YouTube portals in the comments section. It is often attacked by dieticians and laymen who have not tried this diet.

The diet consists of three stages:

a) **Preparation stage** (the most important) **detoxifying the body**, this stage lasts from 2-6 weeks, the first 2-3 days are crucial because we eliminate virtually everything from the diet, leaving only the indicated vegetables and fruits. This is known as prolonged fasting. Indicated products can be consumed in any quantity.

b) Exiting stage, it is divided into weeks,
- in the first week we add all other vegetables and fruits,
- in the second week we add Cereals (including flour products and rice, preferably whole grain), nuts,
- in the third week, dairy (including eggs),
- in the fourth week, meat (starting with fish and lean white meat) and all other products (except forbidden ones - white flour, sugar, yeast, milk - except for fermented products).

c) The stage of the proper diet, the diet is based on vegetables and fruits + meat, fish or poultry, with the elimination of other meat, white flour, sugar, milk (except for fermented products), yeast, alcohol.

In the preparation stage, the following products are allowed: carrots, beets, celery, parsley, horseradish, turnip, radish, various types of cabbage, cauliflower, broccoli, bok choy, kale, Chinese cabbage, arugula, kohlrabi, asparagus, various types of lettuce, spinach, beet leaves, leaf celery, parsley leaves, dandelion, nettle, sorrel, various types of onions, chives, leek, garlic, pumpkin, zucchini, eggplant, cucumbers, tomatoes, peppers and fruits such as apple, grapefruit, lemon. Once a day, you can also eat in decorative amounts (i.e., no more than a handful): berries, kiwi, pomegranate, oranges, tangerines, currants, gooseberries, apricots, watermelons, plums, cherries, raspberries.

Although the diet was created for healing, its main current use is weight loss. Because weight loss is really a side effect, not a goal. Today, it can certainly be said that it is mainly used for weight loss, and predominantly by women.

3.3.1 The Process of Autophagy.

Why exactly does this diet heal? Japanese scientist Yoshinori Ohsumi, who received the Nobel Prize in "Medicine and Physiology" in 2015, answered this question. Actually, Dr. Dąbrowska should have received the award, as she described the mechanisms of autophagy earlier, which is what the Nobel Prize was awarded for.

In a very brief summary - Autophagy is a process in which cells remove and recycle damaged or unnecessary components within the cell to maintain health and function. It is an important repair and regeneration mechanism in many organisms, including humans. Here are a few main mechanisms of autophagy:

- **Formation of autophagosomes**: The autophagy process starts with the formation of a structure called an autophagosome. An autophagosome is a double-membrane vesicle that contains unnecessary or damaged cellular components, such as damaged proteins, damaged organelles (e.g. mitochondria), or other cellular elements.

- **Fusion of autophagosome with lysosome**: The autophagosome then merges with a lysosome, which is a cellular organelle containing digestive enzymes. This fusion creates a structure called an autolysosome.

- **Degradation and recycling of components**: In the autolysosome, lysosomal enzymes digest the content of the autophagosome, breaking down unnecessary or damaged cellular components into smaller molecules, such as amino acids, sugars, and fatty acids. These reduced components can then be utilized by the cell to synthesize new proteins and other components necessary for function.

- **Regulation of autophagy**: The autophagy process is tightly regulated by various factors. Genes that control the expression of autophagy-related proteins play a key role. There are also many signaling pathways, such as the mTOR (mammalian target of rapamycin) pathway, which can inhibit or stimulate autophagy in response to various environmental signals and the state of the cell.

Autophagy plays a significant role in maintaining cellular homeostasis, eliminating toxic components, repairing damage, and regenerating tissues. Disturbances in autophagy mechanisms have been identified as factors associated with various diseases, such as neurodegenerative diseases, cancer, metabolic diseases, and many others.

The fruit and vegetable diet by Dr. Dąbrowska has certain restrictions. It is not recommended for:

- pregnant women,
- during lactation,
- children,
- people with severe depression,
- in case of fear of the diet, which may inhibit self-healing processes.

The fruit and vegetable fasting is also not suitable for people suffering from:
- type 1 diabetes,
- kidney diseases,
- cancer,
- liver diseases,
- anemia,
- cardiovascular and respiratory system diseases
- tuberculosis

- hyperthyroidism
- depression
- anorexia and bulimia

Indeed, it's interesting to consider why Dr. Dąbrowska's diet, given its reported health benefits, is not more widely known and popular. The simple answer to this question is that it's not a profit-driven diet. Therefore, there isn't a strong interest in promoting its wider use.

Interestingly, the diet is also indicated for overcoming addictions. In the first 2-3 days of the preparatory phase, it presents such a shock to the system that the brain is occupied with other problems, shifting its focus away from the addiction.

While Dr. Dąbrowska's diet can have positive health outcomes, it isn't without its drawbacks, especially when applied to men, as I found out personally. However, it's worth noting that despite these shortcomings, the diet can indeed improve health, even in seemingly hopeless situations.

The fundamental issue for men using this diet lies in its calorie content during the preparatory stage. Essentially, the preparatory stage equates to prolonged fasting. Even Dr. Dąbrowska herself mentions that this stage could be replaced by fasting. However, extended periods of fasting can pose health risks and would typically need to be conducted under medical supervision, hence this diet offers a more gentle approach.

Regardless of the quantity consumed, the permitted foods in the preparatory phase will not provide more than 800 kcal. Yet, for normal physiological functioning, men require about 1500 kcal. This discrepancy can lead to temporary impotence. Interestingly, while fasting can enhance sexual potency in women, it reduces it in men. This could pose a problem when a couple decides to undertake the diet together

Moreover, the diet lowers blood pressure and pulse rate, which for a man with already low blood pressure can result in values below normal and an overall feeling of discomfort, something I personally experienced. After the body switches to internal nourishment, between the 2nd and 3rd day, hunger is no longer felt. The body ramps up, with an increase in energy. However, in a negligible number of people, essentially only in men, especially when body fat is not too high, the opposite effect can occur - apathy and weakness, which I also experienced personally.

In conclusion, Dr. Dąbrowska's diet is a great solution in situations of immediate need associated with severe illness. However, for maintaining health or improving it in a slow, gradual process, my own author's diet, which I will discuss in the following chapters, will be much better.

If you are intrigued by this diet and would like to learn more about it, I suggest listening to the lectures available on YouTube by the author herself (simply type into YouTube "dr Ewa Dąbrowska - Lecture part 2"), there is also a part one but it's better to listen to it as a second:

https://www.youtube.com/watch?v=yJn4bf0chxc&t=607s

https://www.youtube.com/watch?v=tFlQXgbi2ns&t=6s

Let me mention that there are books available detailing the diet and a cookbook based on this diet.

3.4 Ketogenic Diet.

The ketogenic diet, also known as the keto diet, is a way of eating that is based on low carbohydrate intake, moderate protein intake, and high fat intake. The goal of the ketogenic diet is to put the body into a state of ketosis, where it primarily uses fats as its main source of energy, instead of carbohydrates.

During a typical diet, the body burns carbohydrates as its primary fuel. However, with the ketogenic diet, by limiting carbohydrate intake, the body begins to produce and use molecules called ketones as an alternative energy source. When the concentration of ketones in the blood rises, the body is in a state of ketosis.

Key principles of the ketogenic diet include:

a) **Low carbohydrate intake**: Limiting carbohydrate consumption is crucial in the ketogenic diet. Typically, it's reduced to around 20-50 net grams of carbohydrates per day, which is a small amount, e.g., in the form of low-carb vegetables.

b) **Moderate protein intake:** Protein intake is moderate in the ketogenic diet to prevent the transformation of amino acids into glucose through a process called gluconeogenesis. It usually constitutes about 20-25% of the total calorie intake.

c) **High fat intake**: Fats are the primary source of energy in the ketogenic diet. They usually make up about 70-75% of the total calorie intake. Natural fats such as plant oils, butter, olives, avocados, nuts, seeds, as well as fatty meats and fish are consumed.

d) **Adequate fiber intake:** Consuming an adequate amount of fiber, primarily from low-carb vegetables, is also important in the ketogenic diet to maintain proper functioning of the digestive system.

The ketogenic diet is used for various purposes, such as weight loss, improving metabolic health, increasing energy and focus, and as an aid in treating certain conditions like drug-resistant epilepsy.

The ketogenic diet has a multitude of proponents, including doctors. It also has a significant amount of critics. In short, its main premise is the consumption of fats, mainly animal ones, while simultaneously consuming about 500 grams of vegetables, including pickles. As one can surmise from the previous sentence, it's not a diet for everyone, because it requires the consumption of large amounts of both meat and vegetables, and there aren't many people who enjoy such a food combination. Unfortunately, the diet won't work if we omit either vegetables or meat.

The basic principles of the ketogenic diet include the consumption of fats and the elimination of carbohydrates, as well as a significant limitation of sugar-containing products such as fruits and vegetables. As part of the keto diet, it is recommended to consume high-fat products such as fatty meats, fish, oils, cream, butter, and nuts. It is important that the fats are of high quality, meaning they are not refined, but only cold-pressed. Especially recommended are olive oil, coconut oil, sesame oil, avocado oil, and coconut butter. In the ketogenic diet, the consumption of avocado as a source of fruit is recommended and the consumption of broccoli, peppers, tomatoes, and cucumbers as vegetables is allowed. You can also consume mushrooms, preferably fried in oil.

The main advantage of the ketogenic diet is the reduction of fat tissue, which contributes to the improvement of the heart, kidneys, and other organs and systems in the body. Additionally, this diet leads to a decrease in blood pressure and a reduction in the levels of sugar, cholesterol, and triglycerides, effectively preventing heart attacks, strokes, and arterial sclerosis. Ketosis has been used in the treatment of drug-resistant epilepsy, especially in children, and also, with appropriate modifications, in the therapy and control of diabetes. Conducted studies also show the beneficial impact of the ketogenic diet on the treatment of Alzheimer's disease, Parkinson's, autism, amyotrophic lateral sclerosis, brain tumors, headaches, and sleep disorders.

After a period of a strict month-long adherence to the diet, when the body has already entered and become accustomed to the state of ketosis, you can introduce a so-called **"cheat day"** once a week, during which you can eat any food, including sweets and sugars. Another advantage of this diet is the beautiful physique it provides, which does not require exercise. For example, the reduction of fat tissue leads to the visibility of abdominal muscles.

An undeniable disadvantage of the diet is the necessity to prepare meals yourself, as ready-made products and dishes available in restaurants and fast food establishments often contain unspecified amounts of sugar. Therefore, during a trip, we cannot just stop at a gas station and eat anything.

Another downside is that extreme sports, like marathons, or continuous exercise exceeding 2 hours, as well as short, intense strength training. Short-term studies show that limiting carbohydrate intake in the diet, leading to reduced glycogen levels, can significantly affect the decrease in exercise capacity, especially in activities where glycolytic-lactate processes predominate. During this type of effort, the body is unable to provide enough oxygen to the muscles to maintain full functioning of aerobic processes. Instead, it uses anaerobic processes such as glycolysis, in which glucose is broken down to produce energy without the involvement of oxygen. Therefore, for athletes, this diet is often modified with so-called carbohydrate loading, which is a complete distortion of this diet.

The third minus is alcohol, which is now much more harmful to health. This happens because ketone bodies are produced in the liver, which significantly burdens it. In addition, alcohol blocks hepatic gluconeogenesis, and often also contains sugar (beer, sweet wine). Therefore, you can drink a small amount of alcohol at a later stage of the diet, for example, on a cheat day.

If you are interested in the topic of this diet - there is a lot of material available in the form of books, websites, studies, and YouTube channels.

3.5 Horsetail Therapy, Plastic and Bisphenol A.

The second half of the 20th century brought many lifestyle diseases that had not previously occurred or occurred only marginally. The cause of this phenomenon is seen in the way of nutrition and environmental pollution. Silicon was eliminated in highly processed food, filtered water also had silicon removed, and food and water storage containers were changed from glass to more practical plastic ones, thus eliminating silicon.

3.5.1 The History of Plastic Creation.

Indeed, the history of plastic is relatively short and began in the mid-19th century with innovations such as parkesine in 1862, the more economically produced celluloid in 1869, and finally the completely synthetic plastic - Bakelite, made from unconventional raw materials, in 1907. Bakelite, named after its creator Leo Baekeland, proved to be an excellent insulating material as it did not conduct electricity.

Plastic production began in 1907 in Belgium. Leo Hendrik Baekeland, a Belgian-American chemist, invented Bakelite, which was the first synthetic plastic to be produced on an industrial scale. Bakelite became a precursor to modern plastics and had a wide range of uses in various fields, including the electronics, automotive, and household industries. From this point on, the production and development of different types of plastics accelerated, and plastic became a commonly used material worldwide.

Plastic started to become a commonly used material worldwide in the second half of the 20th century. The 1950s and 60s saw a rapid development in the plastics industry, which led to the mass production and use of plastics in various areas of life. Plastic was used in packaging production, household items, everyday items, as well as in the automotive, construction, electronics, and many other industries. Its low cost, lightness, durability, and ease of forming contributed to its popularity and widespread use in many areas of life.

3.5.2 Bisphenol A – Lowers Testosterone.

The first mass-produced plastic contained Bisphenol A (currently banned in food packaging production). Bisphenol A (BPA) is an organic chemical compound, whose structure includes two phenol groups. BPA is widely used in the chemical industry as a monomer for the production of polycarbonate and epoxy resins. These materials are commonly used in the production of plastic packaging, bottles, food products, household items, electronic equipment, and many other products.

Bisphenol A is the subject of interest and controversy due to its potential endocrine action. Laboratory studies have shown that BPA can act as a hormone-mimicking compound, affecting the body's hormonal system. There is a concern that long-term exposure to BPA may be associated with various health problems, such as fetal development disorders, reproductive system problems, metabolic disorders, and others.

In response to these concerns, many countries have imposed restrictions on the use of BPA in products intended for food contact, such as baby bottles and food storage containers. Many companies have also taken steps to replace BPA with alternative substitutes with less endocrine potential.

In women, it also causes an increase in testosterone and androstenedione levels, fluctuations in prolactin, and insulin resistance, which is strongly associated with the occurrence of polycystic ovary syndrome PCOS.

Laboratory studies suggest that bisphenol A (BPA) may affect testosterone levels. Some experiments conducted on animals indicate that exposure to BPA may lead to a reduction in testosterone levels. In humans, there is a limited amount of data on the impact of BPA on testosterone levels. Several epidemiological studies suggest that higher concentrations of BPA in the body may be associated with a decrease in testosterone levels in adult men.

3.5.3 Silicon and Its Role in the Body.

Silicon is an essential trace element for the human body, but it is only required in small amounts. Although there is no clear evidence that silicon deficiency is common in healthy individuals, it likely has an impact on the health of connective tissue, skin, hair, and nails. Effects of silicon on the human body:

- **Skin, Hair, and Nail Health**: It is a component of collagen, which is essential for maintaining the elasticity and healthy appearance of these tissues.

- **Bone and Connective Tissue Health**: It plays a role in the metabolism of calcium, magnesium, and other mineral components that are essential for the health of bones and connective tissue.

- **Protection against Free Radicals**: It may act as an antioxidant, helping protect the body from harmful free radicals.

- **Vascular Elasticity**: It may influence the elasticity of blood vessels, which could have a beneficial effect on the cardiovascular system.

„Silicon has the ability to remove from our body aluminum and other heavy metals such as lead, mercury, and cadmium. The accumulation of aluminum in the body is considered a cause of Alzheimer's disease. We live in a time where aluminum surrounds us on all sides - it is in cans, foil, yogurt packaging, pans and pots, grill trays, deodorants, UV filter creams, and processed food.

Fortunately, silicon is our natural shield, protecting us from aluminum and other heavy metals. In the United Kingdom, studies were conducted among people with Alzheimer's disease, which showed that drinking 1 liter of silicon-containing water can accelerate the excretion of aluminum by 70%, and some patients reported clinical health improvement within 12 weeks of therapy.

Silicon is known as the element of beauty. Its delivery with food will provide us with beautiful and healthy hair, skin, and nails. Silicon participates in our body in the production of hyaluronic acid and collagen, providing us with a young and radiant look."[1]

---

[1] https://wodamoda.pl/pijmy-krzem

3.5.4 Horsetail - Silicon Dosag.

The cheapest and most easily accessible form of delivering silicon to the body is dried field horsetail herb. Field Horsetail (Equisetum arvense) is a herbaceous plant belonging to the horsetail family. It is widely distributed in temperate and cool areas worldwide. Field Horsetail is known for its characteristic appearance, resembling reed or brush. The Field Horsetail plant has a stem that is fully green and cylindrical. On the stem, there are delicate, branched twigs, which are covered with scaly leaves. Field Horsetail does not have flowers or fruits. It reproduces through spores that are in characteristic conical spikes at the top of shoots.

Field Horsetail has many uses in natural medicine. It contains many nutrients such as silica, flavonoids, mineral salts, and organic acids. It is used as an ingredient in preparations that strengthen hair, nails, and bones due to its properties that stimulate collagen production and improve the condition of connective tissue. Field Horsetail can also be used as a diuretic, helping to cleanse the body of toxins and excess water.

The herb contains 5-8% silicic acid (including water-soluble silicates) and 1.5% potassium. Flavonoids and trace amounts of alkaloids including nicotine, anti-vitamin B1.

Dried Field Horsetail can be bought on a well-known auction site, for a small amount of money.

How to prepare a decoction of field horsetail: it is recommended to pour three tablespoons of field horsetail herb into 0.75 liters of warm water, then boil it for 15 minutes. After this time, remove the decoction from the heat, set aside for 10 minutes and strain. Drink three times a day, one glass each time. During prolonged use of horsetail extracts, it is recommended to also take Vitaminum B1 tablets 0.003g, 1-2 per day until symptoms of vitamin deficiency subside.

The first therapy with horsetail should be applied for about one month, to be repeated annually for a period of 1-2 weeks.

3.6 Optimal Diet.

Based on my experience with diets and scientific research, I developed my own diet. I wanted it to be as simple and tasty as possible, and I wanted everyone to be able to modify it (within the main assumptions) as needed. This diet can be followed by everyone, and it will also work for people who are not working, those who are working, and those who are on business trips or have irregular working hours.

I personally have been following this diet for 1.5 years, and after the first year of using it, I had full blood diagnostic tests, including morphology, hormones, and mineral levels, and my health is in perfect condition, with my testosterone at the upper level of the norm.

The diet is based on one main meal, which, because it is any meal (a favourite one), will require supplementation. In the diet, we use a feeding window of at least 17 hours. Therefore, the mechanism of autophagy (described in Chapter 3.3 Diet by Dr. Ewa Dąbrowska) is preserved.

Here is an example 24-hour cycle of using the diet - we use the diet every day in the same way, but as needed, we can modify it and slightly change it as needed. The sample day will be presented on a training day (there will be more about training in the following chapters) and with supplementation (which will also be detailed in the following chapters):

- 7:00 We wake up and get up, prepare one apple and two large carrots (you can increase these amounts if needed, but there should not be more than 2 apples), we drink coffee or tea (any kind, just without additions). We can drink the first coffee or tea strong.
- 7:30 7:30 We go to work and are at work before 8:00. At work, until 12:00, we drink more coffee or tea, but this time we drink the coffee very diluted, e.g. a flat teaspoon of instant coffee in 0.5l of water. This process is designed to kill hunger and hydrate the body. After 12:00, we take a break for the

first meal and here we eat the apple and carrot prepared earlier, we can eat at once, we can spread it into portions, depending on the possibilities and needs. Then we move on to drinking, it can be water or tea - preferably green or grain coffee (of course without additives) and so until the end of work. Now remember that we had our first meal after 12:00.

- 16:30 We return home, drink a pre-workout and do a workout lasting about an hour (there will be more about training in the following chapters)

- 17:30 We prepare a meal, here's the good news, it can be any meal, if you like pizza it can be pizza. I buy ready, fresh pizzas from Biedronka (market in Poland), which I season, add a lot of stuffing, raw 1/8 red pepper, raw ½ onion, 100 grams of any sausage, you can also add other additions e.g. pickled cucumber or any product in any configuration. After baking in the oven, which in thermo circulation in an electric stove from room temperature to 180 degrees Celsius takes 8-11 minutes, we add sauces in the form of mayonnaise, ketchup, chili sauce, or any other sauce as desired, sprinkle with granulated garlic. It is important to eat to satiety. At this moment, insulin rush and sleepiness often occur, which unfortunately you have to survive, this is the only downside of this diet. In the first two days, more intense hunger may also occur

- 18:30 About an hour after eating the main meal, we take supplements (those that require eating after a meal - there will be more about supplementation in the following chapters)

- 22:00 We take nighttime supplements, if required

- 23:00 At this time we should accustom the body to fall asleep, which will later happen spontaneously.

It's worth noting here that we can eat pizza every day, it can be a different meal, also eaten daily. It can be a homemade dinner, also two-course, eating in a restaurant, or in any other form. On a training day and when we work full-time, however, we need to be alert or think carefully about the time of the first meal, because having the first meal of the day at a certain time, we should eat the last meal no later than 7 hours after the first meal. That's why it happens to me that I eat the first meal only between 2:00 p.m. and 4:00 p.m. If we work from home or have a job that does not require strict hours, then we have complete freedom. For example, we can start the first meal with the main meal at 2:00 p.m., after 4 hours we will be able to do the training calmly, because most of the food should have been digested. Of course, we take supplements an hour after the main meal. We consume the pre-workout supplement/ shake normally before training, and after training an apple and a carrot.

As you can see from this description, we have freedom and can adapt to the daily requirements of our life cycle.

It may happen that we reach a certain level of weight. Our BMI will be perfectly in the middle of the correct weight, and our weight on this diet will slowly decrease, which we don't want anymore. This may also result from the nature of our work (physical) or the intensity of training. Then we need to slightly change the system and, for example, add a second meal every other day or even daily. However, it should be a slightly different meal, for example, a can of sprats, or smoked sprats (or other fish or poultry) 150 grams with the addition of mayonnaise, or 3 hard-boiled or fried eggs, also with the addition of mayonnaise. However, these dishes do not use carbohydrate additives in the form of bread, potatoes, pasta, rice, or groats. You could say that the second additional meal is a keto meal (chapter 3.4) in a small amount of 150 grams. Of course, the rule of 7 hours between the first and last meal applies.

Sweets are not recommended in the diet, and when we can't resist, sweets should be eaten in small quantities immediately after the main meal, in any case, it is forbidden to consume sweets outside of the 7 hours of meal consumption.

A very good habit is to drink 1 tablespoon of apple cider vinegar, dissolved in a glass of water, before the main meal. It brings many benefits, first of all, it significantly reduces the feeling of hunger, secondly, it regulates blood sugar levels, improves intestinal health, supports weight loss.

Another good habit after the main meal is to drink natural kefir. Kefir is a rich source of B vitamins, such as B1, B12 and folic acid, as well as vitamins K and biotin. Additionally, it provides significant amounts of calcium and magnesium. Kefir also contains essential amino acids, including tryptophan, which has a positive effect on the nervous system and has a calming effect.

Kefir, like pickles, has a hugely positive effect on gut flora and oral bacteria. Many studies indicate that kefir may significantly support the antibiotic treatment of Helicobacter pylori infection (it is estimated that even 70-80% of the Polish population are carriers of this bacterium)

3.6.1 Juice from Celery, Carrots, Apples with Ground Pumpkin Seeds.

For those who have a bit more time and flexibility during the day, I suggest trying to make fresh juice from celery, carrots, and apples with the addition of ground pumpkin seeds around 11:00 a.m. for a period of 4 weeks.

Ingredients: one celery, two apples, and about 250 grams of carrots. At the end, add a large heaping tablespoon of ground pumpkin seeds to the juice. This cocktail excellently cleanses the body and adds a lot of vitamins, which will undoubtedly pay off with visible changes.

Celery juice is a source of vitamin A, vitamins B-2 and B-6, vitamin C, and vitamin K. Additionally, in celery juice you can find:

- Folic acid (vitamin B9): It is essential for the proper functioning of the circulatory and nervous systems and helps in the protection against anemia.
- Pantothenic acid (vitamin B5): It participates in the synthesis of steroid hormones, such as testosterone and cortisol, as well as neurotransmitters and certain vitamins.
- Calcium: It is an important mineral for the health of bones and teeth.
- Potassium: It plays a role in maintaining electrolyte balance in the body and regulates blood pressure.
- Manganese: It is a trace element essential for many metabolic processes.
- Sodium: It is an electrolyte necessary for maintaining fluid balance in the body.
- Magnesium: It plays an important role in many metabolic processes and muscle function.

- Phosphorus: It is essential for healthy bones and teeth, as well as for many metabolic processes.
- Electrolytes: Celery juice contains electrolytes that are important for maintaining body fluid balance and nerve impulse conduction.

Carrot juice is valued for its content of many nutrients, such as:

- Vitamin A: It is a key component for the vision process and maintaining healthy skin.
- B vitamins: They enhance the functioning of the nervous system and contribute to energy production in the body.
- Vitamin C: It speeds up the wound healing process and improves iron absorption by the body.
- Zinc: It aids in the treatment of ulcers and acne, improves the condition of the skin, hair, and nails.
- Phosphorus: It participates in the creation of DNA and maintains the acid-base balance in the body.
- Iodine: It is essential for the production of thyroid hormones, which regulate metabolism.
- Iron: It supports the immune system and is essential for the production of red blood cells.
- Magnesium: It has a calming effect and plays a role in the proper functioning of the cardiovascular system.
- Silicon: It is an important component in building bones and connective tissue.

Additionally, carrot juice has anti-cancer properties, lowers blood sugar levels, reduces cholesterol, improves skin health, and supports the nervous system.

Apple juice is an exceptionally valuable beverage in terms of nutritional value. It is also low in calories (about 46 kcal per 100 g), which is why it is often included in many detoxifying and health diets. Its main advantage is the wealth of vitamins, minerals, and antioxidants. Apple juice is also a source of valuable dietary fiber, which supports digestion and the proper functioning of the intestines.

The most important nutritional components of apple juice are vitamins C, A, E, potassium, and antioxidants. Vitamins C, A, and E play a key role in maintaining health and body function. Vitamin C strengthens the immune system, vitamin A is essential for good vision, and vitamin E is a powerful antioxidant. Potassium is essential for electrolyte balance and the proper functioning of muscles and the cardiovascular system. Antioxidants present in apple juice help fight the action of free radicals, which can cause oxidative stress and cell damage.

Apple juice, as mentioned earlier, can alleviate feelings of hunger. Additionally, it has detoxifying properties, removing toxins from the body and has an alkalizing effect, which contributes to better and faster assimilation of valuable nutrients from both other foods and the juice itself.

Thanks to its detoxifying properties, apple juice can help remove accumulated toxins from the body. Furthermore, its alkalizing action can help restore the acid-base balance in the body, which has a beneficial effect on health.

By detoxifying the body and alkalizing, apple juice creates a favorable environment for the assimilation of nutrients. As a result, both valuable nutrients from other consumed foods and those present in the apple juice itself can be better and more quickly absorbed by the body.

Pumpkin seeds are a rich source of vitamins and minerals that play a significant role in the proper functioning of the body. They contain vitamins E, C, as well as B-group vitamins such as niacin, riboflavin, and thiamine, and also vitamins K and A. Moreover, pumpkin seeds are a valuable source of minerals. They are abundant in zinc, calcium, iron, and magnesium, as well as phosphorus and potassium. It's worth noting that pumpkin seeds also contain monounsaturated and polyunsaturated fatty acids, which have a beneficial effect on the body. Additionally, pumpkin seeds are a source of omega-3 fatty acids and contain large amounts of phytosterols. As a result, pumpkin seeds help lower levels of bad cholesterol (LDL), prevent the development of atherosclerosis, and other lifestyle-related diseases. It should also be emphasized that pumpkin seeds have antioxidant properties, which support the body's functioning and delay aging processes.

Pumpkin seeds are particularly recommended in the diet of men. Thanks to the content of vitamin E, they have a positive effect on fertility, the production, and quality of sperm. It is also worth noting that pumpkin seeds are a rich source of zinc, which plays an important role in maintaining sexual performance.

3.6.2 Healthy Main Course Additions.

Garlic (granulated garlic also has these properties), also known as Allium sativum, is a popular culinary ingredient and has been valued for its health properties for centuries:

- **Heart Health**: It can help maintain heart health by lowering blood cholesterol levels, regulating blood pressure, and improving the elasticity of blood vessels. It can also reduce the risk of developing blood clots and atherosclerosis.

- **Antibacterial and Antiviral Properties**: It contains sulfur compounds, such as allicin, which have antibacterial, antiviral, and antifungal effects. It can help combat various infections, including colds, the flu, and respiratory tract infections.

- **Immune System Support**: It strengthens the immune system, thanks to its antibacterial and antiviral properties. It can help prevent infections and shorten their duration.

- **Antioxidant Properties**: It contains antioxidants, such as flavonoids and vitamin C, which help protect cells from damage caused by free radicals. Antioxidants can help fight inflammation and counteract the aging processes.

- **Anticancer Propertiese**: Research suggests that garlic may have potential anticancer properties, especially in preventing certain types of cancers, such as colon cancer, stomach cancer, and breast cancer. However, further studies are needed to confirm these effects.

- **Antioxidative Properties**: It can help protect cells from oxidative damage. It may reduce oxidative stress and prevent DNA damage.

    Onion, scientifically known as Allium cepa, is one of the most commonly used vegetables worldwide and has many beneficial health properties:

- **Antibacterial and Antiviral Properties**: It contains sulfur compounds, flavonoids, and phytoncides, which have antibacterial, antiviral, and antifungal effects. They can help combat infections, especially those associated with the respiratory system.

- **Immune System Support:** It strengthens the immune system due to the presence of vitamin C, antioxidants, and mineral components. It assists the body in fighting off infections and diseases.

- **Heart Protection:** It may have a beneficial effect on heart health by lowering cholesterol and blood pressure levels. The antioxidants present in it help reduce inflammation and protect blood vessels.

- **Anticancer Properties:** Research suggests that onions may have anticancer properties. The sulfur compounds and flavonoids contained in it may help prevent the development of certain types of cancers, including colon cancer, stomach cancer, and lung cancer.

- **Digestive Support:** It contains fiber, which aids digestion and maintains proper bowel function. Additionally, enzymes present in onions can help with better absorption of nutrients from food.

- **Anti-Inflammatory Properties:** It may help reduce inflammation in the body, especially in conditions such as asthma, rheumatoid arthritis, and bronchitis.

  It's also worth mentioning that onions are rich in vitamins C, B6, manganese, potassium, and antioxidants, which have an overall positive impact on health. They can be consumed raw, boiled, baked, or added to various dishes to enjoy their health benefits.

  Bell pepper, also known as sweet pepper or capia pepper, is a popular vegetable of various colors and shapes. It has many beneficial health properties:

- **High Vitamin C Content**: It is one of the best sources of vitamin C. Vitamin C is essential for a healthy immune system, helps in collagen production, acts as a potent antioxidant, and aids in iron absorption.

- **Antioxidants**: It contains various antioxidants, such as vitamin C, vitamin E, beta-carotene, lutein, and zeaxanthin. Antioxidants help protect cells from oxidative damage, reduce inflammation in the body, and may help reduce the risk of chronic diseases such as heart disease and certain types of cancer.

- **Eye Health Support**: Lutein and zeaxanthin, which are present in bell peppers, are beneficial for eye health. They protect the retina from damage caused by free radicals and light radiation, and may also help prevent macular degeneration and cataracts.

- **Digestive Support**: It is a good source of fiber, which is necessary for proper digestive system functioning. Fiber helps regulate bowel movement, maintain healthy gut flora, and prevent constipation.

- **Low Calorie Content**: It is low in calories, making it a good choice for those maintaining a healthy weight. At the same time, it provides valuable nutrients, such as vitamins and minerals.

- **Anti-Inflammatory Properties**: Nutrients present in bell peppers, such as vitamin C, vitamin E, and antioxidants, have anti-inflammatory actions. They may help reduce inflammation in the body, which can contribute to various chronic diseases.

Bell peppers can be consumed raw, boiled, baked, stewed, or added to various dishes, salads, and sauces. It's important to include different colors of bell peppers in your diet, such as red, yellow, green, and orange, to maximize the diversity of nutrients.

A diet based on the consumption of small fish can provide many health benefits. Here are some health benefits of a small fish-based diet:

- **Source of Healthy Fats**: Small fish such as sardines, herring, mackerel, and anchovies are rich in omega-3 fatty acids, especially eicosapentaenoic acid (EPA) and docosahexaenoic acid (DHA). These fatty acids have beneficial effects on heart health, reducing the risk of cardiovascular diseases.

- **Good Dose of Protein**: They are also a source of high-quality protein, which is necessary for building and repairing tissues in the body. Protein is also essential for maintaining muscle mass, regulating hormones, and supporting immune functions.

- **Abundance of Nutrients**: They are rich in various nutrients, such as vitamin D, vitamin B12, iodine, selenium, iron, and vitamin A. These nutrients play a crucial role in many body functions, such as bone health, immune system, brain function, and vision.

- **Low Risk of Toxins:** They have a shorter life cycle and are lower in the food chain, which means they contain fewer toxins, such as mercury, compared to larger fish. This makes them a safe dietary choice, especially when it comes to pregnant women and young children.

- **Source of Vitamins and Minerals**: Consuming small fish can provide the body with a variety of vitamins and minerals, which are necessary for the proper functioning of the body. For example, sardines are rich in calcium, anchovies provide vitamin E, and herring are a source of vitamin B12.

Free-range eggs are considered better for several reasons. Here are some of the benefits of consuming free-range eggs:

- **Natural Chicken Feed**: Free-range chickens have access to a natural diet, which often includes grass, worms, and insects. This influences the quality of chicken feed and may affect the nutritional composition of the eggs.

- **Nutritional Composition**: Free-range eggs may have a more beneficial nutritional composition compared to eggs from caged hens. According to some studies, free-range eggs may contain higher amounts of vitamins, minerals, and omega-3 fatty acids.

- **Taste Quality**: Due to differences in diet and chicken activity, some believe that free-range eggs have a richer taste and a more intense yolk color.

Mayonnaise, ketchup, and other additives.

It is important to check the composition of food products, such as mayonnaise and ketchup as well as other additives, for several reasons and due to their potential impact on health. Here are some aspects to consider:

- **Nutrients**: Checking the composition of products allows you to identify what nutrients are in the product. You can check the content of fats, sugars, protein, fiber, vitamins, and minerals. Proper understanding of the composition will allow you to better balance your diet and consciously choose products that provide nutritional value.

- **Additives and preservatives**: Many food products, including mayonnaise and ketchup, may contain additives and preservatives. Some of them may be artificial, and some people may be sensitive to certain chemicals. Analyzing the composition will allow you to identify the presence of such additives and make informed decisions about their consumption.

- **Fat, sugar, and salt content**: Mayonnaise and ketchup can be a source of fat, sugar, and salt. Long-term consumption of large amounts of these ingredients can affect health. Analyzing the composition will allow you to assess the content of these ingredients in a given product and choose options that are more in line with your nutritional needs.

- **Allergens**: Checking the composition is especially important for people with allergies or food intolerances. Food product compositions contain information about the presence of potential allergens such as eggs, milk, gluten, nuts, or shellfish. Careful reading of labels will help avoid dangerous ingredients for people with such reactions.

Sometimes we can be surprised by how a cheaper "non-branded" product can be healthier. Let's compare, for example, the popular and well-liked Włocławek (brand in Poland) ketchup (all products available in Poland), which has 23 grams of sugar, and 161g of tomatoes are used to produce 100 grams of the product. In contrast, the inexpensive Biedronka supermarket's "Madero" ketchup stands out for its high tomato content. 232g of tomatoes were used per 100g of ketchup. Sugar is second in the composition, with 20.7g per 100g of ketchup. Similarly, the mayo comparison is underwhelming. The popular Hellmann's mayonnaise - Ingredients: rapeseed oil (76%), water, vinegar, sugar, egg yolk (3%)*, mustard (water, mustard, vinegar, salt, spices, flavors), salt, flavor, color (carotenes), antioxidant (calcium disodium EDTA), *Eggs from litter-raised hens. Compared with Biedronka "Madero" mayonnaise - ingredients: rapeseed oil (79%), water, free-range chicken egg yolk (6%), sugar, spirit vinegar, mustard (water, white mustard, spirit vinegar, salt, sugar), salt, acidity regulator: citric acid, antioxidant: E385. Besides, this is the only cheap mayonnaise that contains free-range chicken egg yolk characterized by a higher content of Omega 3 fatty acids.

4. Supplementation - Essential Dietary Supplement.

Dietary supplementation and training play a crucial role in achieving optimal health and testosterone levels for several reasons: replenishing deficiencies, improving workout performance, speeding up recovery, and optimizing body composition.

I present a list of supplements that may be particularly useful in the process of improving health and testosterone levels in men.

4.1 Supplements in a Man's Diet.

4.1.1 Adek.

This is an abbreviation for vitamins A, D, E, and K - a group of fat-soluble vitamins:

Vitamin A: Supports eye health by maintaining the proper functioning of the retina. It influences the development and maintenance of healthy skin, mucous membranes, and epithelia. It strengthens the immune system. It helps maintain healthy bones.

Vitamin D: Maintains healthy bones and teeth by regulating the absorption of calcium and phosphorus from the digestive tract. It affects the functioning of the muscular and nervous systems. It plays a role in maintaining the proper mineral density of bones. It supports the immune system.

Vitamin E: Acts as a powerful antioxidant, helping to protect cells from damage by free radicals. It influences the health of the skin and hair. It supports the immune system. It has a beneficial effect on heart health by protecting blood vessels from oxidative damage.

Vitamin K: Plays a key role in blood clotting, helping to form clots. It influences bone health by regulating the absorption of calcium and controlling the process of bone mineralization. It may have potential anti-inflammatory action. It is involved in regulating functions beyond the clotting system, such as kidney health and the cardiovascular system.

4.1.2   B Complex.

The B vitamin complex, known as B vitamins or B complex, consists of eight different B vitamins: B1 (thiamine), B2 (riboflavin), B3 (niacin), B5 (pantothenic acid), B6 (pyridoxine), B7 (biotin), B9 (folic acid), and B12 (cobalamin). Here are some important properties of the B complex:

a) **Energy and Metabolism:** B vitamins are essential for the proper functioning of metabolism in the body. They assist in the conversion of nutrients, such as carbohydrates, fats, and proteins, into energy, which is needed to maintain healthy body function.

b) **Nervous System Health**: B complex vitamins play a significant role in the functioning of the nervous system. B6, B9, and B12 are essential for the synthesis of neurotransmitters, such as serotonin, dopamine, and norepinephrine. They aid in maintaining healthy brain function, improve mood, and support concentration.

c) **Skin, Hair, and Nail Health**: Some B vitamins, such as biotin (B7) and niacin (B3), play a vital role in maintaining healthy skin, hair, and nails. They help maintain skin elasticity, promote healthy hair growth, and strengthen nails.

d) **Immune System Support**: Some B vitamins, including folic acid (B9) and vitamin B6, are vital for healthy immune system function. They assist in the production and function of white blood cells, which are key in defending the body against infections.

e) **Heart Health:** Some B complex vitamins, such as niacin (B3), can have a beneficial impact on heart health. Niacin helps maintain healthy cholesterol levels, regulates blood pressure, and supports the proper functioning of the circulatory system.

f) **Red Blood Cell Production:** Folic acid (B9) and vitamin B12 are necessary for the production of red blood cells. They help maintain a healthy hemoglobin level and prevent anemia.

B vitamins are interrelated and enhance each other's action. It is important to maintain a balanced diet that provides an adequate amount of B vitamins.

4.1.3   Beta-Alanine.

This is an amino acid that plays a significant role in the body, especially in the process of carnosine synthesis. Here are some important properties and benefits associated with beta-alanine supplementation:

a) **Increased Endurance and Stamina**: Beta-alanine supplementation can increase carnosine levels in muscles. Carnosine acts as a buffer for acids that accumulate during intense physical exertion. This can help delay muscle fatigue, leading to increased endurance and stamina during high-intensity workouts.

b) **Strength and Muscle Mass Improvement:** It may contribute to an increase in muscle strength and the development of muscle mass. By enhancing workout capacity, it can enable more intense workouts, which can lead to better results in muscle building

c) **Muscle Fatigue Reduction**: It can help reduce the sensation of muscle fatigue that may occur during high-load workouts. It works by reducing the accumulation of lactic acid in the muscles and delaying the onset of fatigue.

d) **Body Composition Improvement**: Research suggests that beta-alanine can influence the reduction of fat tissue and increase muscle mass. This can be beneficial for individuals aiming for fat tissue reduction and body composition improvement.

e) **Antioxidant Properties**: Beta-alanine also exhibits antioxidant action, aiding in the protection of cells from damage caused by free radicals.

It's important to consult with a doctor or a nutrition specialist before starting beta-alanine supplementation. Dosage and individual needs can vary depending on training goals and health condition.

4.1.4   Zinc.

It is an essential trace element that plays many important functions in the body. Here are some important properties and benefits associated with zinc:

a) **Immune System Support**: Zinc plays a key role in the functioning of the immune system. It aids in the production and activation of white blood cells, which are responsible for fighting off infections. A deficiency of zinc can lead to a weakening of the immune system.

b) **Growth and Development Support**: is necessary for the proper growth and development of the body. It is especially important during childhood, adolescence, and pregnancy, when the demand for zinc is increased.

c) **Skin Health**: has a beneficial effect on skin health. It aids in tissue regeneration, soothes skin inflammations, supports wound healing, and can be used in the treatment of acne.

d) **Antioxidant Properties**: Zinc acts as an antioxidant, aiding in the protection of cells from damage caused by free radicals. It helps combat oxidative stress and reduces inflammation in the body.

e) **Cognitive Function Support**: Zinc is significant for the proper functioning of the brain and nervous system. It participates in processes of signal transmission between nerve cells, supports memory, focus, and overall cognitive functions.

f) **Fertility Support**: Zinc plays a crucial role in reproductive health in both men and women. In men, it is necessary for the production of healthy sperm, and in women, it affects fertility and the health of the ovaries.

Zinc is present in many foods, such as meat, seafood, pumpkin seeds, nuts, whole grains, and vegetables. In case of zinc deficiency or special dietary needs, zinc supplementation may be recommended.

4.1.5 D-Asparagine (DAA).

Is an amino acid that may influence the production of testosterone. Studies suggest that DAA supplementation may increase hormone levels in men with low testosterone levels:

a. **Hormonal Regulation**: DAA is involved in hormone regulation in the body, particularly hormones associated with testosterone production. Studies suggest that DAA supplementation may increase testosterone levels in men, leading to improved physical performance, muscle mass growth, and increased libido. However, the results of these studies are mixed, and the long-term effects of DAA supplementation on testosterone levels are still unknown.

b. **Physical Performance**: Some research suggests that D-Aspartic Acid can impact physical endurance and reduce feelings of fatigue. DAA supplementation may influence energy processes in the body, resulting in better performance in high-intensity exercises.

c. **Fertility Improvement**: D-Aspartic Acid might affect male fertility by increasing sperm production. Studies suggest that DAA supplementation may improve sperm motility and semen quality. Further research is needed in this field.

d. **Neurological Functions**: D-Aspartic Acid is present in various brain tissues and is associated with the regulation of neurotransmitters. Some studies suggest that DAA may affect neurological functions, such as memory and focus improvement. However, further studies are needed to confirm these effects.

It's important to note that D-Aspartic Acid supplementation can have side effects and may not be suitable for everyone. Here are some potential side effects that may occur:

a) **Gastrointestinal Disorders**: Some individuals may experience symptoms such as nausea, vomiting, diarrhea, bloating, or stomach discomfort after DAA supplementation. These symptoms may be due to food intolerance or excessive consumption of the supplement.

b) **Hormonal Disorders**: While DAA is involved in hormone regulation, long-term DAA supplementation can lead to hormonal imbalances. This may include changes in testosterone, estrogen, or other hormone levels in the body. Therefore, it's important to exercise caution and monitor your body's response.

c) **Sleep Disorders**: Some individuals report difficulty falling asleep or sleep disturbances after DAA supplementation. This may result from DAA's impact on the nervous system and changes in neurotransmitter levels.

d) **Allergic Reactions**: Some individuals may have an allergic reaction to D-Aspartic Acid. Allergy symptoms can include rash, itching, swelling, or shortness of breath. If any allergic symptoms occur, you should immediately stop supplementation and consult a doctor.

4.1.6 DHEA: Dehydroepiandrosterone.

Is a steroid hormone naturally produced by the adrenal glands and ovaries:

a) **Precursor to Sex Hormones**: DHEA serves as a precursor to sex hormones, such as estrogens and testosterone. It's converted into these hormones in the body. Because of this property, DHEA is sometimes used to regulate the levels of sex hormones in individuals with deficiencies or hormonal dysfunction.

b) **Aging and Skin Health**: DHEA levels in the body naturally decrease with age. Therefore, some studies suggest that DHEA supplementation might have a positive effect on the body's aging process and skin health. However, the results of research in this area are mixed, and the long-term effects of DHEA supplementation on aging and skin health are not fully understood.

c) **Mood and Cognitive Function Improvement**: There's research suggesting that DHEA may have an impact on improving mood, cognitive functions, and memory. However, these results are inconsistent, and the influence of DHEA in these areas is still under investigation.

d) **Libido Enhancement**: DHEA is sometimes used as a supplement to enhance libido and sexual function in individuals with sexual disorders. However, the effectiveness of DHEA in this area is still being researched, and individual effects may vary.

It should be noted that DHEA supplementation can have side effects and may not be suitable for everyone. DHEA is available as a supplement, but it requires a prescription in some countries (it is sold over-the-counter in Poland). Here are some potential side effects that may occur:

a) **Hormonal Disorders**: DHEA is involved in regulating hormones in the body, so long-term DHEA supplementation can impact hormonal balance. This could lead to changes in sex hormone levels, such as estrogens and testosterone, which can have various health consequences.

b) **Skin Effects**: In some individuals, DHEA supplementation can cause acne, skin changes, oily skin, or seborrhea. These side effects are particularly associated with high doses of DHEA.

c) **Sleep Disorders**: Some individuals report difficulties falling asleep or sleep disturbances after DHEA supplementation. This could be related to the effects of DHEA on the nervous system and sleep-regulating processes.

d) **Interactions with Other Medications**: DHEA can affect the metabolism and action of certain medications. It may interact with anticancer drugs, immunosuppressants, antidiabetic medications, and others.

e) **Other Side Effects**: Other side effects may also occur, such as headaches, nausea, changes in cholesterol levels, difficulty urinating, mood changes, changes in body weight, and others. However, side effects can vary depending on the individual and the dose of DHEA.

4.1.7   Glycine.

This is one of the simplest amino acids found in living organisms. In my opinion, it's the best supplement for sleep problems and should be taken directly before bedtime. Additionally, it is one of the three precursors of natural glutathione in the body. Its properties are:

a. **Neurotransmitter and neurological functions**: Glycine acts as an inhibitory neurotransmitter in the brain and nervous system. It is involved in the regulation of muscle tension, cognitive functions, sleep, and mood regulation. Glycine can improve sleep, reduce stress, and improve concentration.

b. **Reduction of stress symptoms:** Glycine is known for its anti-stress properties. Studies suggest that glycine supplementation can help alleviate stress symptoms, reduce nervous tension, and improve well-being.

c. **Improving sleep quality**: Glycine can affect sleep quality by regulating the sleep-wake cycle and reducing the time needed to fall asleep. Research suggests that glycine supplementation can help improve sleep, reduce difficulties falling asleep, and reduce disturbing dreams.

d. **Supporting the immune system**: Glycine plays a role in the functioning of the immune system. It can support regenerative processes, have anti-inflammatory effects, and influence the body's immune response.

e. **Supporting joint and skin health**: Glycine is a component of collagen proteins, which are essential for the health of joints, skin, hair, and nails. It can support tissue regeneration, maintain skin elasticity, and healthy joints.

f. **Other health benefits**: Other health benefits: Glycine may have a beneficial impact on metabolic health, blood sugar regulation, liver health, digestive system, and heart health. However, research in these areas is still ongoing.

4.1.8   Glutathione.

Also known as the tripeptide γ-glutamyl-cysteinyl-glycine, it is an endogenous antioxidant present in living organisms. Here are some facts about glutathione and its potential properties:

a. **Antioxidant**: It is a powerful antioxidant that neutralizes free radicals and other harmful oxidizing substances in the body. It protects cells from oxidative stress and DNA damage, which can contribute to preventing various diseases, including heart diseases, neurodegenerative diseases, and cancers.

b. **Detoxification**: It is a key factor in the body's detoxification processes. The liver uses glutathione to remove toxins such as heavy metals, pesticides, and other chemical substances. Improving glutathione levels can support liver health and overall body detoxification.

c. **Supporting the immune system**: It plays a crucial role in the functioning of the immune system. It helps regulate the immune response, strengthening the immune reaction to infections and diseases. Low glutathione levels can weaken the immune system and increase susceptibility to infections.

d. **Anti-inflammatory properties**: It also demonstrates anti-inflammatory action, assisting in reducing inflammation in the body. Reducing inflammation can have a positive effect on heart health, respiratory system, joints, and overall nervous system function.

e. **Regulation of aging processes:** It is involved in the regulation of the body's aging processes. Its level naturally decreases with age, which can contribute to an accelerated aging process. Supplementation with glutathione or other factors that increase glutathione levels can have a beneficial effect on health and delay the aging processes.

It's important to note that glutathione is produced in the body, and some foods rich in glutathione precursors, such as avocado, broccoli, garlic, and spinach, can help increase its levels. However, glutathione supplementation is also available and can be used to increase the level of glutathione in the body. For the body to synthesize glutathione, the right ingredients and substances are needed

Here are some substances that are essential for the formation of glutathione:

Cysteine: It is a sulfur amino acid and a key component of glutathione. It is synthesized in the body or supplied with the diet. Cysteine is especially important because it contains a thiol group (-SH), which is necessary for the creation of disulfide bridges between glutathione molecules.

Glutamine: This is an amino acid that also plays an important role in glutathione production. It is a precursor to glutamate, which is one of the building blocks of glutathione. It is widely and abundantly found in many foods, so it does not require supplementation.

Glycine: Another amino acid, is necessary for the production of the peptide part of the glutathione molecule. It is the third component of glutathione, alongside cysteine and glutamate.

Vitamin B2 (riboflavin): It is necessary to convert glutathione molecules between their oxidized (GSSG) and reduced (GSH) forms. Increasing the level of vitamin B2 can help maintain glutathione balance in the body.

Vitamin B6 (pyridoxine): It is necessary to convert cysteine into its biologically active form, that is, to convert cysteine into intracellular cysteine.

Selenium: Selenium is a trace element that is important for the activity of enzymes involved in glutathione metabolism. It helps maintain the proper function of glutathione in the body.

All of these components are important for the production and maintenance of appropriate levels of glutathione in the body.

4.1.9   HCA.

Hydroxycitric acid is a chemical compound naturally found in certain plants, particularly in Garcinia cambogia fruits. HCA is a popular ingredient in many dietary supplements marketed as aiding in weight loss. Here are some facts about HCA and its potential properties:

a) **Appetite reduction**: HCA may affect the levels of appetite-regulating hormones such as serotonin. Some studies suggest that HCA supplementation may reduce feelings of hunger and appetite, which can help limit calorie intake and promote weight loss.

b) **Enzyme blocking**: HCA inhibits the action of an enzyme called citrate lyase, which is involved in the process of carbohydrate conversion into fats. By blocking this enzyme, HCA may reduce the amount of fat stored in the body.

c) **Mood improvement**: HCA can affect serotonin levels in the brain, which may have a positive effect on mood and emotions. Increasing serotonin levels may contribute to reducing feelings of stress and improving well-being.

4.1.10 Collagen.

Is a type of protein that is a fundamental component of connective tissue in animal organisms, including humans. It's the most abundant structural protein in the human body and plays a key role in maintaining the health of skin, joints, bones, muscles, ligaments, and connective tissue. Here are some essential facts about collagen:

a. **Structure**: It occurs in the form of long fibers composed of three polypeptide chains, called α-chains. These chains are arranged in a triple helix structure.

b. **Different types of collagen**: There are several different types of collagen, each of which is present in different tissues and serves specific functions. For example, Type I collagen is present in the skin, bones, tendons, and ligaments; Type II collagen is in cartilage, and Type III collagen is in blood vessels.

c. **Structural properties**: It gives connective tissues strength, flexibility, and structure. In the skin, collagen helps maintain its elasticity and resilience while also providing tensile strength. In bones, collagen creates a structure that gives them strength and resistance to fractures.

d. **Regeneration and healing**: It plays a crucial role in tissue regeneration and healing processes. After injuries or damage, the body synthesizes new collagen to repair damaged tissues.

e. **Collagen supplementation**: Because of its significance for the health of the skin, joints, and bones, collagen supplementation has become popular. Collagen supplements may be used to improve skin elasticity, reduce wrinkles, strengthen joints and bones, and support connective tissue health. However, the effects of collagen supplementation are still under scientific investigation, and the results are mixed.

It's important to note that collagen is a large protein that isn't entirely absorbed by the body after consumption. However, collagen supplementation can provide the body with the amino acids necessary for collagen synthesis within the body.

4.1.11   Fenugreek.

Fenugreek, also known as Trigonella foenum-graecum, is a plant from the Fabaceae family. It has a long history of use in folk medicine and is widely used both as a spice in the kitchen and as a medicinal herb. Here are a few details about fenugreek and its potential health properties:

a) **Blood Sugar Regulation**: is known for its impact on blood glucose levels. Studies suggest that fenugreek can help regulate blood sugar levels, which can be beneficial for individuals with type 2 diabetes.

b) **Digestive Aid**: may have a positive impact on the digestive system. It is often used in traditional medicine to alleviate stomach ailments such as heartburn, bloating, and constipation.

c) **Lactation Improvement**: Fenugreek is often used as a natural remedy to support milk production in breastfeeding women. Research suggests that fenugreek consumption can increase the amount of milk and improve the quality of mother's milk.

d) **Heart Health Support**: Fenugreek can have a positive effect on heart health by reducing levels of cholesterol and triglycerides. Research suggests that regular consumption of fenugreek may help lower the risk of cardiovascular diseases.

e) **Immune System Support**: Fenugreek is rich in many nutrients, such as vitamins, minerals, and antioxidants, that can support immune system health and protect the body from infections.

Clinical trials indicate that supplementation with fenugreek extract can affect the increase in blood testosterone levels in men. According to these studies, positive effects were observed when using fenugreek in the form of capsules at a dose of 250-500 mg per day for a period of 8-12 weeks. The level of free testosterone increased by as much as 47%.

4.1.12   Creatine.

This is an organic chemical compound that naturally occurs in animal organisms, including human organisms. It is synthesized in the liver, kidneys, and pancreas from amino acids such as glycine, arginine, and methionine. Creatine plays a key role in delivering muscle energy, especially during intense physical exertion. Here are some facts about creatine and its properties:

a) **Improvement of endurance and muscle strength**: Creatine is commonly used as a dietary supplement by athletes and physically active individuals because it can contribute to an increase in endurance and muscle strength. Creatine supplementation may help increase the production of energy in muscles, which translates into improved athletic performance, especially in short-term, intense efforts.

b) **Water retention in muscles**: Creatine can cause water retention in muscles, which may lead to weight gain. This phenomenon is sometimes desired by individuals seeking to increase muscle mass and strength.

c) **Muscle recovery**: Creatine can accelerate the process of muscle recovery after training, reducing the feeling of fatigue and supporting energy renewal.

d) **Creatine in the brain**: Studies suggest that creatine may have a beneficial effect on cognitive functions and brain health. It may support memory, concentration, and the level of mental energy.

4.1.13 L-Carnitine.

This is an organic chemical compound that plays a crucial role in the body's energy metabolism. It is naturally produced in human bodies and also occurs in some foods:

a) **Fat acid transport**: it plays a key role in transporting fatty acids to the mitochondria, where they are used as an energy source. It assists in converting fatty acids into energy, which is important for maintaining proper fat metabolism.

b) **Weight loss and fat burning**: Due to its role in fat metabolism, L-carnitine is often advertised as a supplement supporting weight loss and fat burning. Some studies suggest that L-carnitine supplementation may influence increased fat oxidation and improved physical performance, but the results are mixed.

c) **Reduction of fatigue**: it may contribute to reducing the feeling of fatigue and improving physical performance. This may be particularly beneficial for people with an L-carnitine deficiency, such as older people, athletes, or individuals with certain conditions.

d) **Support for the cardiovascular system:** it plays a role in maintaining the health of the cardiovascular system. It assists in energy production by the heart, improves blood flow, and may influence the reduction of the risk of certain heart diseases.

e) **Improvement of brain function**: Some research suggests that L-carnitine may have a beneficial effect on cognitive functions and brain protection. It may influence the improvement of concentration, memory, and mood.

f) **Muscle health support**: it may have a beneficial effect on muscle health, supporting regeneration, reducing muscle damage after intense physical effort, and reducing the risk of muscle acidification.

4.1.14   Magnesium.

It is one of the essential trace elements that are necessary for the proper functioning of the body. It is involved in many physiological processes and plays a significant role in human health:

a) **Bone structure and bone health**: Magnesium plays a crucial role in the metabolism of calcium and vitamin D, which affects bone health. It is necessary for calcium absorption and maintaining the proper bone structure. A deficiency in magnesium can contribute to bone weakening and an increased risk of osteoporosis.

b) **Muscle function:** Magnesium plays an important role in muscle functioning. It is necessary for proper muscle contraction, including the heart muscle. A deficiency in magnesium can lead to muscle cramps, muscle spasms, and muscle weakness.

c) **Regulation of the nervous system**: Magnesium affects the functioning of the nervous system, assisting in the regulation of nerve conduction and neurotransmission. It may contribute to reducing symptoms of stress, anxiety, and improving sleep quality.

d) **Blood sugar level regulation**: Magnesium is involved in glucose and insulin metabolism. It may help in maintaining proper blood sugar levels and reducing the risk of type 2 diabetes.

e) **Supporting the immune system**: Magnesium plays a role in the functioning of the immune system and inflammatory processes. It may support the body's immune function and prevent inflammatory conditions.

4.1.15   NAC.

N-acetylcysteine is a derivative of an amino acid called cysteine. It has many potential health benefits and is used both as a dietary supplement and a drug:

a) **Liver protection**: NAC is known for its liver-protective properties. It is used in the treatment of paracetamol overdose as it helps neutralize its toxic effects on the liver. NAC may also support liver health in the case of liver diseases such as liver cirrhosis or viral hepatitis.

b) **Antioxidant activity**: NAC is a powerful antioxidant that helps neutralize the action of free radicals and protect cells from oxidative stress. It may support the health of the respiratory system, the cardiovascular system, and prevent cell damage caused by free radicals.

c) **Lung health support**: NAC may be useful in treating some lung diseases such as chronic bronchitis or obstructive lung disease (COPD). It helps to thin and cough up mucus, which may facilitate breathing and reduce symptoms.

d) **Cognitive function improvement**: NAC may have a positive impact on cognitive functions such as memory, concentration, and cognitive ability. Research suggests that NAC may be beneficial in cases of neuropsychiatric disorders such as Alzheimer's disease, schizophrenia, or obsessive-compulsive disorder (OCD).

e) **Kidney health support**: NAC may have a beneficial effect on kidney health. It may help protect the kidneys from damage caused by toxic factors or urinary system diseases.

4.1.16   CBD Oil.

CBD oil is a product that contains cannabidiol (CBD), one of the main compounds found in hemp. CBD is one of many plant compounds known as cannabinoids. Here are a few details about CBD oil and its properties:

a.   **Stress and anxiety relief**: CBD is known for its potential anti-anxiety and stress-relieving properties. It may help in reducing symptoms of anxiety, such as restlessness, tension, or sleep disorders.

b.   **Pain and inflammation reduction:** CBD has analgesic and anti-inflammatory actions. It may help alleviate pain of various origins, including neuropathic pain, joint pain, or migraines. In addition, CBD may aid in reducing inflammatory states in the body.

c.   **Sleep quality improvement**: Some studies suggest that CBD may help improve sleep quality and alleviate sleep disorders, such as insomnia or stress-related sleep disorders.

d.   **Nervous system health support:** CBD has the potential to influence the nervous system and neurotransmission. It may have a beneficial effect on cognitive functions, memory, and brain health. Some studies also suggest that CBD may have neuroprotective action, protecting nerve cells from damage.

e.   **Epilepsy counteraction**: CBD is one of the few cannabinoids that have been approved by the US Food and Drug Administration (FDA) for use in treating certain types of epilepsy. It has been found that CBD can reduce the frequency of epileptic seizures in some patients.

4.1.17   Omega-3.

Omega-3 fatty acids, such as EPA (eicosapentaenoic acid) and DHA (docosahexaenoic acid), are essential for heart and brain health. Research also suggests that omega-3 supplementation may help increase testosterone levels in men.

Omega-3 is a type of polyunsaturated fatty acids that are essential for the proper functioning of the body. These are fats that the body cannot produce on its own and therefore must be supplied externally, through diet or supplementation:

a) **Heart Health:** They play a significant role in maintaining heart health. Studies suggest that regular consumption of omega-3s can help lower blood triglyceride levels, regulate blood pressure, reduce the risk of blood clots, and improve the lipid profile. They may also help reduce inflammatory processes in blood vessels.

b) **Brain Health**: They are important for proper brain development and function. They are associated with improved cognitive function, concentration, memory, and mood. Studies also suggest that they may play a role in protecting against neurodegenerative diseases, such as Alzheimer's disease and dementia.

c) **Inflammation Reduction**: They have anti-inflammatory properties, which may contribute to reducing inflammatory states in the body. They can help alleviate symptoms of arthritis, asthma, inflammatory bowel diseases, and other inflammatory conditions.

d) **Skin Health**: They play a role in maintaining healthy skin. They can help moisturize the skin, reduce psoriasis, acne, and other skin problems. In addition, they have a protective action for the skin against the harmful effects of UV radiation.

e) **Mood Regulation**: They may have a beneficial effect on mood regulation. Some studies suggest that omega-3 supplementation can help alleviate symptoms of depression, anxiety, and bipolar affective disorders.

Omega-3 sources are primarily fatty sea fish, such as salmon, tuna, herring, and sardines. They can also be available in the form of supplements, such as fish oil or algae for people who prefer vegetarian or vegan options.

4.1.18   Selenium.

Selenium is a trace element that is essential for the body in small amounts. It has many important functions and health properties:

a) **Antioxidant action**: Selenium acts as a component of antioxidant enzymes, such as glutathione peroxidase, which help neutralize the harmful effects of free radicals in the body. As a result, it can protect cells from oxidative damage.

b) **Immune system support**: Selenium plays a vital role in the functioning of the immune system. It aids in the production of antibodies, which are crucial in fighting infections, and can influence the activity of immune system cells.

c) **Thyroid health**: Selenium is essential for the proper functioning of the thyroid. It aids in the synthesis of thyroid hormones and can influence their metabolism in the body. Selenium deficiency can lead to thyroid disorders, such as hypothyroidism.

d) **DNA protection**: Selenium may have a beneficial effect on protecting DNA from damage. It can assist in repairing damaged DNA and maintaining its integrity.

e) **Heart health**: Some studies suggest that selenium may have a beneficial effect on heart health. It can aid in lowering cholesterol levels, regulating blood pressure, and reducing the risk of cardiovascular diseases.

Selenium is naturally found in many foods, such as Brazil nuts, seafood, meat, eggs, sunflower seeds, and whole grain cereals. Selenium dietary supplements are also available. However, it is important to moderate and not exceed the recommended daily dose of selenium, as too much can be harmful to the body.

4.1.19   Tribulus terrestris.

This is a plant that has long been used as a means to improve male potency. Studies suggest that supplementation with tribulus terrestris can increase testosterone levels in some men.

Tribulus terrestris, also known as puncture vine, is a plant that has various potential properties:

a) **Enhancement of sexual functions**: It is often advertised as a substance that can improve sexual functions. There is a hypothesis that it may increase testosterone levels, which could contribute to enhancing libido and sexual performance. However, research results on this matter are mixed, and the effect of Tribulus terrestris on sexual functions remains a subject of debate.

b) **Improvement of physical endurance**: It is sometimes used as a supplement that may support the increase in strength and physical endurance. Some studies suggest that it could enhance the production of nitric oxide, which can lead to the dilation of blood vessels and improve blood flow to the muscles, potentially contributing to increased physical endurance. However, research results on this matter are contradictory.

c) **Anti-inflammatory and antioxidant properties:** It contains certain compounds that exhibit anti-inflammatory and antioxidant actions. This may help protect cells from oxidative damage and prevent inflammatory states in the body.

d) **Support of urinary system health**: It is sometimes used in traditional medicine to support the health of the urinary system. It may help alleviate symptoms associated with urinary bladder infections or kidney stones.

4.1.20   Vitamin B2.

Riboflavin is essential for energy conversion and metabolism. A deficiency of this vitamin can affect the production of testosterone. Riboflavin supplementation can contribute to maintaining an adequate hormone level. It plays an important role in the body, and its properties and functions include:

a) **Energy metabolism**: it is essential for the proper metabolism of carbohydrates, fats, and proteins. It participates in the processes of converting these substances into energy, which is needed by the body to function properly.

b) **Protection against oxidative stress**: it acts as an antioxidant, which means it helps to neutralize harmful free radicals in the body. It protects cells from oxidative damage and prevents cell aging.

c) **Supporting skin health**: it is important for skin health. It can help maintain healthy skin, prevent inflammatory skin conditions such as acne, and support the wound healing process.

d) **Supporting eye health**: it plays a role in maintaining healthy eyes. It is necessary for the production and regeneration of the retinal pigment, which is essential for proper vision. A deficiency of vitamin B2 can lead to vision problems such as light sensitivity or tired eyes.

e) **Production of red blood cells**: it is essential for the proper production of red blood cells. It participates in the process of creating and maintaining healthy blood cells, which affects the transport of oxygen and nutrients to all tissues of the body.

Vitamin B2 is naturally present in many foods, such as dairy, meat, fish, nuts, seeds, whole grains, and leafy vegetables. If you are unable to provide enough vitamin B2 in your diet, you may consider supplementation.

4.1.21 Vitamin B12.

Also known as cobalamin, it is one of the B group vitamins that are essential for the proper functioning of the body:

a) **Support of the nervous system**: it plays a crucial role in the functioning of the nervous system. It is essential for the production of myelin, a substance that surrounds nerves and contributes to improved nerve conduction. A deficiency of vitamin B12 can lead to nerve damage and neurological symptoms such as tingling, muscle weakness, or coordination problems.

b) **Production of red blood cells**: it is essential for the production of red blood cells. It supports the creation and maturation of erythrocytes, which transport oxygen to the body's tissues. A deficiency of vitamin B12 can lead to anemia, characterized by fatigue, weakness, and pale skin.

c) **Homocysteine metabolism**: it is part of enzymes that metabolize homocysteine, a harmful chemical compound present in the blood. High levels of homocysteine in the body can increase the risk of cardiovascular disease. Vitamin B12 helps convert homocysteine into other safe compounds, affecting cardiovascular health.

d) **Supporting brain health:** Vitamin B12 plays a significant role in brain and nervous system functioning. It can affect cognitive functions, memory, concentration, and mood. A deficiency of vitamin B12 can be associated with neurological symptoms such as memory disorders, depression, or mood disorders.

e) **Absorption and metabolism of other substances**: Vitamin B12 is essential for the proper absorption of folic acid, which is important for DNA production and healthy cell growth. Moreover, vitamin B12 is also vital for the metabolism of amino acids and fats.

Vitamin B12 naturally occurs in animal products such as meat, fish, eggs, and dairy. It is also available as a supplement, especially for people on vegetarian or vegan diets, who may have difficulty getting enough vitamin B12 from their diet.

4.1.22   Vitamin C.

Also known as ascorbic acid, it is one of the most well-known vitamins with powerful health properties:

a) **Strengthening immunity:** it plays an important role in the functioning of the immune system. It aids in the production and activation of white blood cells, which are key to fighting infections. Additionally, vitamin C may help to shorten the duration and alleviate symptoms of the common cold and flu.

b) **Strong antioxidant action:** it is a powerful antioxidant that helps neutralize free radicals in the body. It protects cells from oxidative damage, prevents cell aging, and supports the regeneration of other antioxidants, such as vitamin E.

c) **Support of collagen production:** it is essential for the production of collagen, which is a key structural protein in the skin, connective tissues, bones, blood vessels, and many other parts of the body. Vitamin C supports wound healing, the maintenance of skin elasticity, and a healthy appearance.

d) **Supporting heart health**: it can have a beneficial impact on heart health. It acts as an antioxidant that helps protect blood vessels from oxidative damage. Vitamin C may also help lower LDL cholesterol (bad cholesterol) levels and regulate blood pressure.

e) **Iron absorption:** it enhances the absorption of iron from food, which is particularly important for individuals with iron deficiencies or those suffering from iron deficiency anemia. Consuming vitamin C in combination with iron-rich foods can improve the absorption of this nutrient.

Vitamin C naturally occurs in many fruits and vegetables, such as citrus fruits, kiwi, bell peppers, strawberries, berries, broccoli, and spinach. Vitamin C supplements are also available in various forms, such as tablets, capsules, or powders. However, it is important to consult a doctor before starting vitamin C supplementation, especially in the case of any illnesses or interactions with other medications.

4.1.23   Vitamin D.

Vitamin D deficiency is often associated with reduced testosterone levels. Vitamin D supplementation may help regulate hormone levels. Additionally, vitamin D plays a crucial role in maintaining overall health and strengthening the immune system.

Vitamin D is an important nutrient that performs many vital functions in the body:

a) **Bone health support**: One of the main functions of vitamin D is to support bone health. It assists in the absorption of calcium and phosphorus from food, which is necessary for maintaining strong and healthy bones. Vitamin D deficiency can lead to bone weakening and increased risk of osteoporosis.

b) **Regulation of calcium levels in the blood:** it helps maintain a balance of calcium levels in the blood. It assists in absorbing calcium from the intestines and controls its release from bones to maintain appropriate calcium levels in the blood. Calcium is essential for many processes in the body, such as muscle contractions, nerve functioning, and blood clotting.

c) **Supporting the immune system:** it also affects the immune system. It aids in regulating the body's immune response, supporting healthy immune system function. Vitamin D deficiency can affect immunity weakening and increase susceptibility to infections.

d) **Impact on mental health:** Some research suggests that vitamin D may have a positive impact on mental health, including mood regulation and reducing the risk of depression. However, the mechanism of action in this area is not fully understood and requires further research.

e) **Impact on heart health:** There is research suggesting that adequate levels of vitamin D may be associated with a lower risk of cardiovascular diseases. Vitamin D may affect blood pressure regulation, inflammation reduction, and blood sugar control, which may contribute to heart health.

Vitamin D is produced by the body in response to the sun's rays on the skin. It can also be consumed in the diet, in products such as fatty fish (e.g., salmon, tuna), vitamin D fortified milk, egg yolks, and in the form of supplements. It's important to maintain appropriate vitamin D levels in the body, and in the case of deficiency or doubt, it's advisable to consult a doctor to determine the right dose of supplementation.

4.1.24   ZMA.

This stands for "Zinc-Magnesium Aspartate," a dietary supplement that contains a combination of zinc, magnesium, and vitamin B6. Here are a few details about ZMA and its potential properties:

a. **Supporting testosterone production**: ZMA is often advertised as a supplement that affects the increase in testosterone levels. Zinc is an essential mineral for testosterone production, and magnesium and vitamin B6 may have a beneficial effect on hormonal function. However, there is a limited amount of research confirming these effects.

b. **Supporting muscle recovery**: Zinc, magnesium, and vitamin B6 play an important role in the process of muscle recovery after intense physical exertion. They can help reduce fatigue, support healthy sleep, and affect metabolic processes related to muscle recovery.

c. **Improving sleep**: ZMA may have a beneficial effect on sleep quality. Magnesium and vitamin B6 are involved in the processes regulating the body's circadian rhythm and the production of sleep-related hormones, such as melatonin. ZMA supplementation may contribute to better sleep and overall rest.

d. **Supporting immune function**: Zinc is an essential component for the proper functioning of the immune system. It can affect strengthening immunity and protecting the body from infections.

4.1.25   Swedish Herbs.

Swedish herbs, also known as "bitters" or "Swedish elixir", are a mixture of herbs and plant substances macerated in alcohol. They have a long history of use in folk and traditional medicine, and their recipe is attributed to the Swedish botanist and doctor, Dr. Samuel Hahnemann.

The composition of Swedish herbs can vary depending on the manufacturer, but typically they contain a combination of herbs such as:

Chamomile (Matricaria chamomilla)

- Oak bark (Quercus robur)
- Green mint (Mentha spicata)
- Sage (Salvia officinalis)
- Cinnamon bark (Cinnamomum verum)
- Fennel (Foeniculum vulgare)
- Field horsetail (Equisetum arvense)
- Comfrey bark (Symphytum officinale)
- Ginseng (Panax ginseng)

In Poland, the most popular version is Swedish Herbs with wormwood according to Maria Treben - containing a composition of herbs: wormwood, myrrh, saffron, senna, rhubarb root, turmeric root, manna, theriac, angelica root, elecampane root, camphor.

Swedish herbs are recommended for both prophylactic purposes, aimed at strengthening the body's immunity, and for medicinal purposes, in case of various ailments and diseases.

Swedish herbs are valued for their properties alleviating skin problems such as acne, rashes, burns, frostbite, and aiding the healing process of scars.

Additionally, they can help reduce muscle, joint, and rheumatic pain. Swedish herbs are also recommended as a remedy for menstrual pain, toothache, migraines, sore throats, fever, chills, and help with various types of infections and inflammations.

A ready-made mix of herbs can be purchased on a popular auction portal.

Preparation method:

The herbs should be poured over with 1.5 liters of 38-40% alcohol.

- Then leave the mixture for 14 days in a warm place at a temperature of about 25 degrees Celsius.
- It is important to shake the mixture every day.
- After 14 days, strain the mixture and transfer it to dark bottles.
- The bottles should be tightly closed and stored in a cool place.
- Such a prepared tincture can be stored for several years.

Consume 1-3 tablespoons, add to half a glass of water, drink before sleep.

4.2   Supplementation Rules.

General rules for supplementation:

- **Proper supplement selection**: Choose supplements from reputable manufacturers and check their composition, quality, and safety.
- **Dosage**: Follow the dosage recommendations given on the supplement package or the doctor's advice. Do not exceed the recommended doses unless your doctor advises it.
- **Regularity and long-term use**: Supplementation works effectively when it is continued regularly over a long period of time. Expected results may take time, so it is important to use supplements systematically according to recommendations.
- **Be aware of interactions**: Some supplements may interact with medications or other supplements.
- **Monitor your body's reactions**: Be aware of your body and observe how it reacts to supplementation. If there are any adverse side effects or unusual symptoms, consult a doctor.
- **Do not replace a healthy lifestyle**: Remember that supplements should not replace a healthy lifestyle, which includes a proper diet, regular physical activity, adequate sleep, stress reduction, and avoiding addictions.
- **Test levels**: Detecting deficiencies, monitoring toxicity, individual needs, optimization, progress assessment.

It's worth remembering that an excess of most vitamins and minerals can be harmful to health. Vitamin A and iron are examples of this. Another issue is dosage selection. There are men who weigh just under 70 kg, while others may weigh over 140 kg. For substances like creatine, it's very easy to determine the right dose - you simply use a multiplier of 0.5 g of creatine for every 10 kg of body weight. Things become much more complicated with vitamin D. This vitamin is extremely important in the bodies of children, women, and men. The dosage of vitamin D is generally measured in internationally accepted units (IU). For example, for most countries, the daily norm for infants is set at 400-1000 units, while for men over 70 it's 800-1000 units. So, for a child weighing 3 kg and a man weighing 100 kg, the vitamin D dose can be identical despite a 33-fold weight difference. In Poland, the Dietary Supplement Committee operating under the Sanitary-Epidemiological Council has stated that the safe dose of vitamin D is a maximum of 2000 IU (50 µg) per day.[2] Interestingly, scientific research and associated recommendations suggest that obese individuals (BMI >30) should take double doses, i.e., up to 4000 units per day.[3] Dr. Hubert Czerniak presents an interesting standpoint. He claims that the supplementation of vitamin D should be between 20,000 and 50,000 units per day, but it should be combined with vitamin K2 MK7 at a dose of 100-200 micrograms (mcg). According to him, you cannot take high doses of vitamin D alone. Hubert Czerniak is known for his media appearances on the subject of vitamin D intake, where on camera he can drink 100,000 units of vitamin D at once. He also refers to the textbook by Professor Wojciech Kostowski "PHARMACOLOGY. BASIC

---

[2] https://www.poradnikzdrowie.pl/zdrowie/leki/witamina-d-dawkowanie-u-niemowlat-dzieci-i-doroslych-normy-spozycia-aa-yyxn-M1dp-csoV.html

[3] https://dietetykanienazarty.pl/b/witamina-d3-przedawkowanie-najlepsze-dawkowanie

PHARMACOTHERAPY. MANUAL FOR MEDICAL STUDENTS AND DOCTORS. VOLUME 1 AND 2", where the indicated daily norm is 10,000 units of vitamin D per kg of body weight. It's easy to calculate that for a man weighing 100 kg, the indicated daily dose in such a case should be 1 million units.[4]

Another issue in determining the correct doses of a given substance and its levels in the blood is the low repeatability of studies in some areas of medicine and establishing norms, as mentioned in Chapter 3.1 Diet, which will ruin your life. Blood sugar levels can serve as an example.

Blood sugar level norms may vary depending on countries and medical organizations. Additionally, these values can change over time as measurement methods and understanding of the significance of blood sugar levels have evolved over the years.

At the end of the 20th century, for example, the American Diabetes Association (ADA) defined a normal fasting glucose level as a value below 110 mg/dl (milligrams per deciliter). Values above this threshold but below 126 mg/dl were considered pre-diabetic, a state called impaired fasting glucose. A fasting blood sugar level of 126 mg/dl or higher was the criterion for diagnosing diabetes. Today, the norm is considered to be fasting (before eating) - blood sugar levels should range from 70 to 99 mg/dL (3.9 to 5.5 mmol/L). Interestingly, in the early 1960s, the normal fasting blood sugar level was often defined as below 140 mg/dl.

---

[4] https://www.youtube.com/watch?v=rkf6ONzm-Js

4.2.1   Most Common Side Effects of Supplementation.

The side effects of dietary supplementation can vary depending on the type of supplement, dosage, length of use, and individual characteristics of a person. Here are some of the most common side effects that can occur with supplementation of various substances:

- headaches,
- nausea,
- loss of appetite,
- fatigue,
- muscle cramps,
- diarrhea,
- bloating,
- abdominal pain,
- anxiety,
- insomnia,
- tachycardia,
- high blood pressure

We can thus talk about a certain wisdom of our body, which signals that a given substance is harmful to us or is already in our body in an optimal amount, and its additional intake can cause harm. Therefore, it is worth introducing individual supplements into the diet one by one and observing the body's response. In the event of any negative symptom, it is recommended to eliminate the given supplement. From my experience, the most common side effect is abdominal pain.

Often with long-term supplementation, it is difficult to determine what is causing a given side effect. In such cases, it is necessary to discontinue all supplementation and reintroduce supplements individually or in groups, starting with safer ones like vitamin C. Some substances, like creatine, should not be taken on an empty stomach because they will cause stomach pain in the long run. Then it's enough to move their intake to after the main meal.

What's interesting is that a given supplement can cause a side effect that is very individual. For example, the previously mentioned creatine, when consumed on an empty stomach, causes some people to have abdominal pain the next day after consuming red wine (this dependency does not apply to other alcohols). In such unusual cases, it is often difficult to establish a direct cause-effect relationship.

According to medical practice, before starting any vitamin or mineral supplement, we should test its level in the blood (probably privately, as it would be hard to get such tests from a doctor - public health service, especially when it would involve a large number of tests) and then consult a doctor who would assess the need for supplementation and its dosage for a certain period of time, followed by a subsequent control test. This procedure would be very costly, as for example, the cost of testing the level of selenium in the blood is about PLN 100, and determining the level of Glutathione, although it is performed in a small number of facilities, costs about PLN 140. As you can see, these are not inexpensive things.

4.2.2   Supplementation of Children up to 15 years old.

Supplementation for children may be important in certain cases, however, the decision to introduce it should always be consulted with a pediatrician or dietitian.

Below are a few basic rules you should know about supplementation in children:

- **Balanced diet**: In most cases, children should get all the nutrients they need from a balanced diet. Supplements are usually recommended only when a child's diet is unable to provide all necessary nutrients, which could be the result of certain health conditions or specific diets (e.g., vegetarian, vegan, eating disorders).

- **Vitamin D:** In many countries, including Poland, vitamin D supplementation is recommended for children from the first days of life, due to its key role in the development and maintenance of healthy bones. However, dosing should be adjusted to the child's age and health condition.

- **Vitamin B12 and Omega-3**: Children on a vegan or vegetarian diet may need additional supplementation with vitamin B12 and Omega-3, which are often difficult to obtain from a diet without animal products.

Remember that an excess of certain vitamins and minerals can be harmful, so it's important to always consult the decision about supplementation with an appropriate specialist. Additionally, the quality of supplements can vary greatly, so it's always worth choosing products from trusted manufacturers.

Now for the facts. Children usually have a selective diet, to which it's very difficult to introduce any supplement, an example might be difficulties with swallowing. Children's diet often comes down to huge amounts of carbohydrates, with the omission or exclusion of meat. In such a case, it will be necessary to supplement vitamin B12 as needed - since it is very safe, there is little risk of side effects, and the tablets themselves are very small and virtually tasteless. Another important supplement will be ADEK, which is also available in liquid form with a dropper dispenser and is easy to adjust to the child's weight. It will be more difficult to introduce vitamin C, due to its sour taste, however, there are also versions for children in a slightly sweetened taste. Omega 3 in capsules is very easy to swallow, you can also replace pure Omega 3 acids with cod liver oil in capsules, where you will also find all ADEK ingredients. Once every 1-2 weeks, it's worth providing Zinc and Selenium (in the daily dose for adults), but each time you need to observe if the side effects mentioned in section 4.2.1 occur. Other supplements should not be given to a child as a preventive measure.

4.2.3   Supplementation of Young Men Aged 15-29.

The supplementation of young men aged 15 to 29 does not have to be exorbitant and it really comes down to a few essential supplements. The cheapest and most effective solution would be to purchase a complete set called "**Olimp Vita-Min Multiple Sport Mega Caps® - 60 Capsules**". The set consists of 30 capsules of vitamins and 30 capsules of minerals. As you can easily deduce, it lasts for a whole month, and its cost is not too high - around 30 PLN. The downside to this solution is the entire range of vitamins and minerals without specific supplementation, and the number of supplements in this set is impressive:

- Vitamin A 800 µg
- Vitamin D 10 µg
- Vitamin E (mg α-TE) 24 mg
- Vitamin C 290 mg
- Thiamine (vit. B1) 19.4 mg
- Riboflavin (vit. B2) 19.6 mg
- Niacin (mg NE) 31 mg
- Vitamin B6 18 mg
- Folic acid 400 µg
- Vitamin B12 23 µg
- Biotin 100 µg
- Pantothenic acid 12 mg
- Citrus bioflavonoids 100 mg
- Artichoke extract (5% cynarin) 80 mg
- Pumpkin seed extract 5:1 60 mg
- Common nettle extract 60 mg
- Green tea extract 55% EGCG, including 3-gallate (-) epigallocatechin 60 mg
- ALA (alpha-lipoic acid) 10 mg

- Black pepper extract (95%) BioPerine® 1 mg
- Magnesium 190 mg
- Calcium 100 mg
- Potassium 75 mg
- Zinc 15 mg
- Iron 3 mg
- Manganese 1.8 mg
- Copper 0.5 mg
- Iodine 150 µg
- Chromium 150 µg
- Selenium 75 µg

The above set can also be used every other day. Adding every day:

- **Vitamin D** 2000 IU (50 µg)/day / for obese men, dose x2,
- **Vitamin C** 500 mg - best to buy 1000 mg tablets (not capsules) and break in half,
- **Omega 3 Acids** 1000 mg / day,
- **Creatine** 0.5g per every 10kg of weight/day after the main meal - creatine should not be taken on an empty stomach,

+ in case of sleep disorders
- **Glycine 3g** directly before sleep,
- **CBD oil 40%** number of drops adjusted empirically,

+ before training
- **Beta-Alanine** 3g,
- **HCA** 350 mg + **L-Carnitine** 350 mg.

4.2.4　Supplementation of Men Aged 30-39 lat.

Supplementation for men from 30 years of age must already be more comprehensive and comes down to a wider list of supplementation, after the main meal:

- **ADEK** in tablets, composition (Vitamin A 800 μg, Vitamin D 50 μg / 2000 IU, Vitamin E 12 mg, Vitamin K 75 μg),

- **B Complex composition** (Vitamin B3 16 mg, Vitamin B5 6 mg, Vitamin B6 1.4 mg, Vitamin B2 1.4 mg, Vitamin B1 1.1 mg, Vitamin B9 200 μg, Vitamin B7 50 μg, Vitamin B12 2.5 μg),

- **Zinc** 15 mg,

- **DDA** 3000 mg, in one serving before bed – a side effect may be sleep disturbance, in this case it should be discontinued,

- **DHAE** 50 mg – a side effect may be sleep disturbance, in this case it should be discontinued,

- **Collagen** 2200 mg, systematically taken, the dose can be reduced to 500 mg / day,

- **Fenugreek extract** 600 mg,

- **Creatine** 0.5g per 10 kg of body weight/day after the main meal - creatine should not be taken on an empty stomach,

- **Magnesium** 400 mg - should be taken in two doses during the day,

- **NAC** 100 mg,

- **Omega 3 acids** 1000 mg,

- **Selenium** 200 µg,

- **Tribulus terrestris** 500 mg,

- **Vitamin B12** 500-700 µg, after a monthly period of saturating the body, you can switch to 500-700 µg once a week,

- **Vitamin C** 500 mg - it's best to buy 1000 mg tablets (not capsules) and break them in half,

- **Vitamin D** 2000 IU (50 µg)/day,

- **Glycine** 3g directly before sleep - sleep regulation

    + in case of sleep disorders:

- **CBD oil 40%** number of drops adjusted empirically,

    + before training:

- **Beta-Alanine** 5g,

- **HCA** 350 mg + **L-Carnitine** 350 mg.

Please note that in this case we have permanently introduced Cysteine (NAC - L Cysteine) and Glycine, the two most important precursors for the body to produce Glutathione. "Glutathione deficiency can lead to many abnormalities, among which oxidative stress is the most dominant - a common ailment of our times. Oxidative stress is the cause of many serious diseases, including cancer and age-related disorders such as Alzheimer's and Parkinson's. Alcohol abuse, improper nutrition, too much processed food, medicines and other substances of abuse are large doses of oxidants, with which the body, especially the liver, cannot cope. Glutathione reduces the amount of these oxidants (free radicals), protecting cells and mitochondria from damage and the development of inflammation. As a result, it prevents the fatty degeneration of liver cells. It can also slow down the aging process, improve concentration and skin appearance, support better sleep and increase body endurance. In addition, it supports the immune system, playing an important role in the functioning of lymphocytes."[5]

---

[5] https://www.zeberka.pl/pielegnacja/glutation-i-zagrozenia-zwiazane-z-jego-niedoborem/

4.2.5 Supplementation of Men Aged 40+ years.

Supplementation for a man from the age of 40, after the main meal:

- **ADEK** in tablets, composition (Vitamin A 800 µg, Vitamin D 50 µg / 2000 IU, Vitamin E 12 mg, Vitamin K 75 µg),

- **B Complex composition** (Vitamin B3 16 mg, Vitamin B5 6 mg, Vitamin B6 1.4 mg, Vitamin B2 1.4 mg, Vitamin B1 1.1 mg, Vitamin B9 200 µg, Vitamin B7 50 µg, Vitamin B12 2.5 µg),

- **Zinc** 15 mg,

- **DDA** 3000 mg, in one portion before sleep - a side effect can be sleep disturbance, in this case it should be completely discontinued,

- **DHAE** 50 mg – a side effect can be sleep disturbance, in this case it should be completely discontinued,

- **Glutathione** 500-1000 mg

- **Collagen** 2200 mg, systematically taken the dose can be reduced to 500 mg / day,

- **Fenugreek extract** 600 mg,

- **Creatine** 0.5g per every 10kg of weight / day after the main meal - creatine should not be taken on an empty stomach,

- **Magnesium** 400 mg - should be taken in two doses during the day,

- **NAC** 100 mg,

- **Omega** 3 fatty acids 1000 mg,

- **Selenium** 200 µg,

- **Tribulus terrestris** 500 mg,

- **Vitamin B12** 500-700 µg, after a monthly period of saturating the body, you can switch to 500-700 µg once a week,

- **Vitamin C** 500 mg - it's best to buy tablets (not capsules) 1000 mg and break in half,

- **Vitamin D** 2000 IU (50 µg)/day,

- **Glycine** 3g directly before sleep - sleep regulation

  + in case of sleep disturbances

- **CBD Oil 40%** the number of drops adjusted empirically,

  + before training

- **Beta-Alanine** 5g,

- **HCA** 350 mg + **L-Carnitine** 350 mg.

In the case of a man aged 40+, Glutathione has been permanently added due to the fact that after the age of 45, the body's natural production of Glutathione dramatically decreases. Unfortunately, Glutathione is very poorly absorbed from the gastrointestinal tract, most of it is digested, only the remnants that manage to get to the intestines. The best solution in this case are capsules. There is also an intravenous version of Glutathione called TAD 600, but this solution is very expensive and requires medical handling. Therefore, it seems a better solution to provide smaller amounts of this substance orally every day. Interestingly, in Italy, TAD 600 is very popular and when cancer markers are detected, doctors first apply therapy with this drug, and most often it is the only effective way to fight cancer. Therefore, it can be said that Glutathione, which is little known and popular in Poland, is number one when it comes to human health.

It is also worth mentioning the problem of the eyes here, which after the age of 40 affects virtually everyone sooner or later. They have become popular due to our increased time spent in front of computer screens, smartphones or tablets. The blue light emitted by these devices can contribute to digital eye fatigue and disrupt the sleep cycle. Glasses with a blue light filter can help minimize these effects, especially for people who spend many hours in front of the screen.

5. Power in Action, Success in Training.

If you've made it this far, congratulations – you've taken the last step to transforming yourself into the best version of you. But remember, the journey doesn't end with reading this book. This is just the beginning of your path to self-improvement. What really counts is how you apply the knowledge gained in your daily life.

In this chapter, I've attempted to create a training plan that will serve both beginners and experienced athletes. Although each of us is different and requires an individual approach to training, I recommend certain basic principles here that are universal and can help you achieve your goals. If you take sport seriously and it has been part of your life for years, you probably won't find much in this chapter, especially if you are in top form.

Firstly, training should primarily be a pleasure. Many of us tend to approach sport as a task that must be done, but the truth is that if you don't enjoy it, it will be harder for you to maintain regularity. That's why I always recommend finding an activity that you are passionate about. If there isn't one, you need to develop a habit, but to develop this habit, you need a workout that won't torment you every day. Only one that will leave you wanting more.

Secondly, remember that it's not all about intensity. It is often better to focus on the quality of the training, not the quantity. A well-planned, moderate-intensity workout can yield better results than endless hours of exhausting exercise.

Finally, regardless of age, weight, or experience, remember the necessity of proper nutrition. What we eat has a huge impact on our ability to achieve results in training. Whether you're just starting your physical activity journey or you're an experienced athlete, proper nutrition is the key to health and success. Only after reaching some basic level can you modify both the diet and the form of training, but you have to start somewhere.

These are just the basic principles that can help you on your way to becoming the best version of yourself. Remember, everyone is different and what works for one person may not necessarily work for another. Therefore, it's important to listen to your body and adjust your workout to your individual needs and goals. Exercise is supposed to make you healthy, you don't have to achieve better and better results, you don't have to compete with anyone, unless it makes you happy or helps you achieve your GOAL.

Let's start with the fact that any extreme is bad and everything in excess is harmful. Therefore, in my opinion, it's hard to talk about health in the context of professional sport but this book does not pertain to that.

5.1 Doctor's Recommendations Regarding Training Intensity.

The recommendations for the amount and intensity of workouts can vary depending on a person's age, physical fitness level, health status, and goals. Below are general guidelines that are usually recommended for most healthy adults:

- **Moderate-intensity aerobic training**: The World Health Organization (WHO) recommends at least 150 minutes of moderate aerobic activity each week. This could include activities such as brisk walking, cycling, swimming, dancing, or even housework that raises your heart rate.

- **High-intensity aerobic training**: An alternative to 150 minutes of moderate activity could be 75 minutes of intense aerobic activity weekly. Intense aerobic activities include running, intense stationary cycling, jumping rope, or high-intensity interval training (HIIT).

- **Strength training exercises**: Additionally, the WHO recommends conducting strength training exercises involving major muscle groups at least twice a week. This can include strength training using weights, resistance exercises like yoga or Pilates, or even bodyweight exercises such as push-ups or squats.

- **Physical activity and sedentary lifestyle**: It should also be remembered that prolonged sitting, even if you exercise regularly, can have a negative impact on health. Therefore, it is recommended to take regular breaks during the day, which would involve walking, stretching, or short exercises.

Remember, however, that these recommendations may not be suitable for everyone, especially if you have any health problems or have not been active before. In such cases, it's always worth starting with shorter forms of training. For many people, starting with short exercise sessions and gradually increasing their intensity and duration can be a good approach. Remember, any physical activity is better than no activity at all.

5.2 How to Start, or the Beginning of Activity.

As I wrote earlier, the assumption of my training proposal is to make it as easy, cheap, and accessible as possible. If you want to allocate additional resources to it, that's great. For some people, this will be motivation - because if they spend money on a personal trainer or a gym membership, they will not want to waste this money by not using it. On the other hand, for those who do not have additional resources, the expenditure on a personal trainer will be impossible, and this will be their "excuse" when it comes to starting activities. The situation is similar when it comes to training with someone else - shared with another person. For one person, this will be additional motivation, because once you arrange a training session, it will be harder to give it up. On the other hand, if one of the people training together loses their enthusiasm, the other will be completely devoid of motivation.

Using a paid gym membership can also be a problem in itself. You need to set aside more time for training, because you need to get to the gym. People's activities usually look similar, so people who work a nine-to-five job will want to use the gym after work, and these places will be more crowded in the afternoon, which may make it difficult to train on specific machines.

Personally, I'm not a fan of paying for physical activity, certainly not in a recreational version or for health maintenance. It's worth introducing healthy habits that cost nothing but will improve our energy balance in and of itself. Therefore, we should change the way we think about our training. We can actually throw out the word training and replace it with an unnamed habit - which becomes an integral part of our life.

You can achieve this in a simple way, starting from the analysis of the individual possibility of changing your activity and then adapting/modifying it to the transformations in our life.

I will try to give examples in a moment, which will guide you, the reader, to a plan of daily activity tailored to your needs. Of course, it is not possible to take into account all individual cases, because each of us leads a different life, but it will allow you to analyze the introduction of changes in your life. It is also important to look at your specific case in terms of opportunities, not problems. If you assume from the start that you won't make it, you're assuming failure from the start, not even giving yourself a chance.

First, from the chapter on supplementation, I'll remind you about so-called pre-workouts. Pre-workouts, also known as pre-workout supplements, are dietary supplements consumed before training to increase the body's endurance and improve the effectiveness of exercises. The formulas of these products usually contain various ingredients aimed at increasing energy, endurance, strength, and concentration. The most known / cheap and generally used is caffeine, which is found in coffee. Another cheap and proven substance is creatine, which has the advantage that it can be consumed at any time of the day - but it should be consumed only after a meal. However, the most spectacular pre-workout, in my opinion, is beta-alanine, it gives a noticeable increase in desire, endurance, and strength. Beta-alanine also has a specific effect, which people taking it describe in different ways, it's "skin burning", "skin itching", for some people it's unpleasant and described as painful. Let me just add that you can regulate this effect by the amount of substance taken. Over time, the body gets used to it and the effect is no longer so noticeable. Beta-alanine is a proven substance, considered safe, also giving a "mental kick". You can read more about this in the chapter on supplementation. I would just like to add that in my opinion it is better to invest in supplementation than in a personal trainer.

If you are a young obese man or a senior man, your advantage will be free time and the ability to adjust your diet, supplementation, sleep, physical activity to your needs. The downside is probably a lack of larger resources. However, physical activity does not really require any financial input. The most expensive in this case will be supplementation, and this can be planned for months. If you have never had anything to do with planned activity, a walk is enough to start with :D However, we will modify this walk a bit. You should plan it every other day for 40-60 minutes. Physical exertion should be carried out for over 30 minutes, as endorphins are produced after this time, and we then talk about the so-called feeling of euphoria. For this walk, we will need a stopwatch or a smartphone - a mobile phone is common today, and it has a stopwatch function, in an android phone press clock, then switch to the hourglass sign - set the timer for one minute. Now, starting the walk, we go at a normal pace for a minute, and then a fast march for the next minute, and so alternating for the set time of 40-60 minutes.

Summary: we implement an optimal diet and supplementation, start systematic physical activity in the form of minute intervals, walk / fast march. In the beginning, we do the required blood tests and possible treatment.

We get the body used to it for 1-3 months. After this period, we change our activity into just a 40-minute march, if possible we increase the time to 60 minutes. We are not interested in distance at all, we can go out of the building and go fast for 30 minutes, then we go back home. The next stage will be jogging / march intervals, also alternating every minute. After another 1-3 months, a 40-minute jog will be possible and we stay on this activity, moving on to optimal training, which will be discussed later in the chapter. Please note that the only parameter we are interested in is time, it's about putting strain on the heart during this time.

If we work full-time and the distance to work is not far, let's say the distance is up to 5 km, we also plan our activity during the journey to work. We don't use a car, we do a "workout" but we do it very loosely going to work, whereas from work analogously we try a fast march or even a jog, it depends on our overall condition.

It may also happen that for certain reasons, we will not be able to run. An example could be a nagging knee injury, then we need to look for other activities: cycling, swimming (by the way, swimming is definitely the best activity, as it engages almost all parts of the body). Of course, we can choose any sport that gives us joy, such as table tennis, in which case we need equipment and a partner. We should also, as far as possible, give up driving a car. Go shopping more often, using a backpack. Visit family and friends on foot. I know that this may not always be possible, for example due to time constraints, but moving on foot (not on an electric scooter or public transport) should be our default option.

When our BMI reaches the norm. There are applications available on smartphones to calculate our BMI, for example, in the Android system, the "BMI Calculator" app, the BMI standard is 18.5 to 25

5.3 Optimal Training.

As we already know, testosterone is a hormone that plays a key role in regulating many functions of the body, including muscle development, red blood cell production, libido, and mood. One way to naturally increase testosterone levels is through regular physical activity. Here are a few types of exercises that can help:

• **Strength Training:** Studies have shown that strength training - such as weight lifting - is one of the most effective ways to increase testosterone levels in men. Try to work all the major muscle groups, with different weights and varying intensity.

• **High-Intensity Interval Training (HIIT)**: High-intensity interval workouts can also boost testosterone levels. These exercises usually involve short, intense periods of activity, interrupted by short rest periods.

• **Endurance Training**: Long-distance running, cycling, swimming, and other forms of aerobic exercise can also help raise testosterone levels, although not as effectively as strength training or HIIT.

If we already have a base in the form of condition for longer training, we can now remodel it a bit. In the free version, we only use a smartphone. It has a lot of great free apps for home workouts. Exercises that use body weight are a great way to work out at home, as they do not require special equipment. Moreover, the weight is always adapted to our capabilities, which significantly reduces the possibility of injury.

A recommended free app, available for android smartphones is an application called "Home Workout - No Equipment". When launching the app, we enter basic data: gender, age, weight and take a short test to determine our level of advancement.

Later, we set the training plan, as the first one I suggest "Whole Body Challenge 7x4" in this training plan we determine the number of days in the week in which we want to exercise. I recommend working out 3 times a week. As needed, you can do them more or less often. After the workout, we get a question about the selection of training intensity. Whether the training was just right, too strong, too weak. Then a question whether to increase the intensity of the training, decrease it or leave it unchanged. I recommend not to go crazy at the beginning and not to increase the intensity too quickly, as I wrote earlier. It's better to be under-trained than overtrained.

The app offers amazing possibilities. Thanks to it, we can train individual parts of the body: abdomen, chest, arms, legs, shoulders and back at intensity: beginner, intermediate and advanced. For us, the legs will be the most important, because that's where the largest muscles are, and exercising large muscles increases testosterone the most. Each body part is important, so we should try to train all muscles symmetrically.

If we have a correct BMI (within the norm), then after the body workout (at the beginning it lasts only 15-20 minutes) we do running training directly. However, in this case at a distance of about 3 km. The aim is to maintain endurance and condition, while extending the training to 40 minutes.

If someone likes to run, you can do body training one day and go running for 40 minutes the next. Personally, I like this activity, I often use the "reader" app in this case, which allows you to read books in PDF format. Interesting reading motivates me to run longer. It's also worth running "around town", on different routes. We have here an additional mobilization effect, because after reaching a certain place we have to return, even if we don't feel like it :D We should also adopt the rule that daily running workouts should not be longer than 8 km. Unless you're preparing for a goal, like finishing a marathon. Such goals are surprisingly not easy to achieve. They require long planned trainings, proper running shoes, which we replace after a certain number of kilometers - this is due to the loss of shoe cushioning. And above all, the workouts should take place on a professional surface, because city concrete is not suitable cushioning for our legs in a run. Just preparing for a marathon requires expert knowledge. It should also be noted that this type of activity (marathon running or very long distances) can be associated with a decrease in testosterone.

Training using your own body weight may be adequate for many people, however, if you aspire to achieve significant results, especially in terms of body aesthetics, it is worth considering regular exercise in a professional fitness center. In such context, using the services of a qualified personal trainer or independent in-depth training techniques could be recommended, as an incorrect approach to exercise can bring more harm than benefits, potentially resulting in long-term health problems. However, we will not discuss the details of proper gym exercises in this compendium, as there are many specialized publications on this subject, which are available for those interested.

At one point, I decided to introduce an innovative approach to physical activity, which in my opinion is an attractive alternative to monotonous exercises. I bought a full-face swimming mask - "Subea Easybreath 500", also available in the Decathlon store, on a renowned auction portal. I also purchased a buoy-backpack, thereby increasing safety during long-distance swimming sessions.

The functioning of the mentioned mask keeps our body on the surface of the water, even when we are motionless. The tube, located above the water surface, allows for free breathing, and if necessary, you can use the buoy and hold it during rest.

On the first day of using this set, I was able to swim 3 kilometers, even though I hadn't been swimming for many years. This set has many advantages, such as the ability to pack your things and dive into the water in one place, and then exit at any other, with all items and clothes safely stored in the backpack. My personal record is 3 hours of swimming without a break.

Unfortunately, the limitation of this solution is our geographical location, which allows us to use this kind of attraction only in the summer season.

In the further part of this chapter, I would like to present a few more interesting ideas for improving health, which are indirectly related to workouts.

5.3.1 Muscle Rolling.

Loosening muscles with a massage roller, also known as muscle rolling or foam rolling, is a self-massage technique that uses various tools such as massage rollers, lacrosse balls, tennis balls, or special massage sticks to mimic the effects of sports massage. On a well-known auction site, just type the phrase "rolling pin". The most useful for us will be a large smooth roller without any protrusions and a small ball, a set is sold with another addition of two merged small balls (I personally do not use it).

Below are some basic body rolling techniques:

- Rolling push-ups: Apply the weight of the upper body to the massage roller, starting from the chest. Do a few slow push-ups, moving the roller up and down.
- Thigh rolling: Sit on the massage roller and move it up and down your thighs, from your hips to your knees.
- Calf rolling: Sitting on the floor, place the roller under your calves and move it up and down.
- Back muscle rolling: Lying on the floor, place the roller under the lower part of the back and move it up and down.
- Shoulder muscle rolling: Standing facing a wall, place the roller between the body and the wall and move it up and down the shoulder muscles.

Remember that muscle rolling should not cause extreme pain. It should be comfortable and bring relief. If you feel severe pain during rolling, consult a physiotherapist. Rolling should be done at a very slow pace, it should be slow rolling aimed at relieving muscle tension. Tight muscles can be painful, you can feel that after the roller goes over a certain tight point, we feel pain that gradually subsides. It is also important to avoid rolling directly on joints and bones. Focus on muscles and soft tissues.

Muscle rolling can help relax tense muscles, improve mobility, and relieve post-workout muscle pain. It's worth incorporating it into your workout routine both before and after training.

On YT, we will find a lot of material regarding rolling specific parts of the body:

https://www.youtube.com/watch?v=kHXg7klo7zM

5.3.2 Cold Showers.

Some time ago, I visited an osteopath. Interestingly, this specialty is not recognized by some doctors in our country or they simply lack knowledge about it. An osteopath is an expert in the field of osteopathy. The training process - to acquire this specialization, is detailed and requires intensive education. Initially, it is necessary to obtain a degree in medicine or physiotherapy through a five-year master's program. The next step is to complete an additional five years of osteopathic studies. After completing this stage of education and passing the clinical examination, this person qualifies to practice as an osteopath. Such an advanced level of education is required because specialists in this field must have a holistic, comprehensive approach to understanding musculoskeletal anomalies and the general dynamics of body functioning.

During the visit, the doctor convinced me to take cold showers. Although in my case, cold water was my Achilles' heel and I never thought that anyone would persuade me to this kind of "pleasure".

Cold water showers, also known as cold showers, are a form of hydrotherapy and can bring many health benefits. Below I describe the process of using cold water showers and the benefits they can bring:

Process:

- **Start with a warm shower**: Start with a moderately warm shower that will allow you to relax and cleanse your skin.

- **Gradually lower the temperature**: Slowly lower the water temperature to give your body time to adjust to the cold water. You can start with cold water on your legs and gradually raise it.
- **Make it short**: You don't have to spend a lot of time under a cold shower. Even a short, 30-second cold water shower can be beneficial.
- **Repeat daily**: Regularity is key to reaping the benefits of cold water showers. Try to make it part of your daily routine.

Benefits:

- **Improved circulation**: Cold water causes the blood vessels to contract, which helps speed up blood circulation. This in turn can help reduce swelling and bruising.
- **Boosting the immune system**: Studies have shown that regular cold water showers can increase the number of white blood cells in the body, which are key to the immune system.
- **Increased energy**: Cold water can have a stimulating effect, increasing energy levels and alertness.
- **Improved mood**: Some studies suggest that cold water can contribute to the release of endorphins, which are called "happiness hormones". It can help improve mood.
- **Recovery after exercise**: Cold water showers are popular among athletes as a way to speed up recovery after intense training, as they can help reduce post-exercise muscle pain. However, remember that we do not take cold showers immediately after training. Sudden contact of a heated body with cold water can lead to thermal shock.

5.3.3 The Last Issue - Good Sleep.

What ends our day and ensures the regeneration of strength is sleep, this inconspicuous, yet indispensable element of a healthy lifestyle. The last issue of this chapter concerns sleep - an issue that cannot be overestimated in the context of men's health and the regulation of testosterone levels.

Sleep is not only a rest time for our mind, but also for our body. During sleep, tissue regeneration takes place, including muscle tissue, which was strained during training. It is then that our body begins to repair the micro-injuries that occurred during intense physical activity, allowing for muscle growth and development.

Sleep is also essential for our mind. During sleep, the brain processes and stores the information we received during the day. It is during sleep that our brain "charges the batteries", so that we can function effectively the next day.

However, sleep has yet another, extremely important function, especially for men - it is during sleep that our body produces the most testosterone. Testosterone is a hormone that is necessary for the proper functioning of a man's body. It regulates, among other things, libido, muscle mass, energy levels, and even mood.

Therefore, the requirements for sleep are a minimum of 7-8 hours per day. The reader may ask - what if I sleep less? Here we come to worrying data. Research shows that when we sleep only 6 hours a day, testosterone levels can drop by up to 15%. If this time is shortened to 5 hours, the level of testosterone may already drop by over 30%.

These are alarming statistics that show how important sleep is for men's health. Neglecting an adequate amount of sleep can lead to a significant decrease in testosterone levels, which in turn has a negative impact on our health, well-being, and overall quality of life. Therefore, sleep should be treated as one of the foundations of a healthy lifestyle, on a par with a good diet, regular physical activity, and appropriate supplementation.

6. Conclusion.

Summary and Conclusions

The journey I have taken you on through these pages not only shows the diversity and complexity of health problems men can encounter, but also the wealth of solutions available to each of us. Each chapter of this book contains tools that can be applied in practice, and their regular use leads to lasting changes.

Remember, the key to health lies not in one specific aspect - nutrition, exercise, supplementation, or stress management - but in the integration of all these aspects. Your lifestyle as a whole plays a key role in your health, and health is the foundation for good quality of life, full of energy, satisfaction, and longevity.

Each of us is different, and what works for one person may not work for another. That is why it is so important for every man to have access to solid knowledge and tools that will help him understand and improve his health, taking into account his unique needs and conditions. This book has been created to provide you with these tools and help you understand how to use them in practice.

Health is not a goal to be achieved, but a process that requires constant commitment and attention. Just as regular physical exercise strengthens muscles, so regular care for health strengthens our ability to cope with daily challenges and stresses. It is an investment that brings measurable benefits over a lifetime.

I encourage you to approach health as a journey that is unique to you. Use this book as a guide that will help you find your own path to health and well-being.

Remember, your health is your most precious resource. Take care of it every day. You deserve it.

www.ingramcontent.com/pod-product-compliance
Lightning Source LLC
Chambersburg PA
CBHW070944260726
48661CB00003B/1109